A MANUAL
FOR WRITERS

*of Term Papers, Theses,
and Dissertations*

A MANUAL
FOR WRITERS
of Term Papers, Theses, and Dissertations

THIRD EDITION, REVISED

By

KATE L. TURABIAN

THE UNIVERSITY OF CHICAGO PRESS

CHICAGO AND LONDON

Library of Congress Catalog Card Number: 67–20252

THE UNIVERSITY OF CHICAGO PRESS, CHICAGO 60637

The University of Chicago Press, Ltd., London W. C. 1

Third Edition, Revised, published 1967

Fourth Impression 1969

Printed in the United States of America

Foreword

This manual is designed to serve as a guide to suitable style in the presentation of formal papers—term papers, reports, articles, theses, dissertations—both in scientific and in non-scientific fields. While the ideas, the findings, and the conclusions put forth in the paper are of primary importance, their consideration by the reader depends in large measure upon an orderly presentation, well documented and free of mechanical flaws.

In the main, the manual is addressed to the writers of the papers, who have the major responsibility for the organization and form in general. The section on typing is addressed especially to the typists, who have the responsibility for preparing the final copies; much of that section, which deals with the mechanics of typing, may be of no interest to the writers, unless it be to those who expect to prepare their own final typescripts. Professional typists, and secretaries who now and again are called upon to whip into shape a report in which only the bare facts are ready for presentation when it reaches their desks, may well find the greater part of the manual useful in their task.

It must be pointed out that no suggestions are given here about *how to write*. The assumption is that, if the writer feels the need of further training in composition, he will consult a reliable up-to-date work on English composition.[1]

In general, the style here recommended is that of the University of Chicago Press as set forth in *A Manual of Style* (11th ed., 9th printing; Chicago: University of Chicago Press, 1964) and exhib-

[1] One may be mentioned: Porter G. Perrin, *Writer's Guide and Index to English* (3d ed.; Chicago: Scott, Foresman & Co., 1962).

ited in its publications, both books and scholarly journals. In some
scientific fields the specific form of literature citation used by a leading journal in a field not covered by periodicals issued by the University of Chicago Press is recommended. Although not all areas in
scientific fields are represented in the examples cited, in their main
outlines the examples illustrate the various accepted usages in scientific writing.

I am greatly indebted to the University of Chicago Press for its
generous cooperation in making this publication possible. Two former members of the staff I would mention especially: Miss Mary D.
Alexander, who was Production Editor during my years at the University as Dissertations Secretary, taught me the first rudiments of
bibliographic style and gave ready answers to many a thorny question that plagued me from time to time. The late Morton Grod-
zins, Professor of Political Science and at one time Editor of the
Press, gave me the courage to undertake the first revision and expansion of this manual. And again it is the influence and participation
of the Press that have induced me to embark in this further revision.

I had some ideas in reserve and sought more from former students
at the University and from others who teach and are long-time users
of the manual. The expansion of the sections on quotations and on
punctuation—the first particularly with respect to ellipses—was suggested by Geoffrey Plampin, the present Dissertations Secretary,
as well as by several others. Aware of the heavy schedules carried
by present-day students, I looked for ways to lighten the task of
preparing formal papers. Two may be mentioned: Combining the
examples of footnote citations each with its corresponding bibliographic entry is a step toward immediate clarification of their differences that I believe should be a great time saver. And the single
recommendation of the short-form title for secondary references,
where the current manual offers choices, is a straightforward han-
dling of the problem that should reduce appreciably the time spent
in checking and rechecking of footnotes. The current *Manual of*

Style takes into consideration "changes in literary practice and new decrees of learned societies and of library associations" (*A Manual of Style*, 11th ed., 9th printing, p. v), and those which bear upon the content of this small manual are reflected in it.

The contributions made to the first revision by Miss Winifred Ver Nooy, formerly Reference Librarian of the University of Chicago Libraries, are carried over in different form in the section on public documents.

Being obliged to look for a new library home, I have found one of great warmth and goodwill in the Stanford University Libraries, where the same knowledgeable, imaginative, and generous help is accorded to me as that so long enjoyed at the University of Chicago.

All the suggestions and the aid received from the various sources here mentioned have been valuable. If they have been poorly acted upon in any instance, the responsibility is mine alone. But of course my hope is that the best of which I am capable may continue to be of service to the users of this little book.

K. L. T.

MENLO PARK, CALIFORNIA

Contents

I

Format of the Paper

1. Normally, a paper[1] is made up of three main parts: the front matter or preliminaries, the text, and the reference matter. In a long paper each of these main parts may consist of several sections (see below); but in a short paper there may be nothing more than a title page and text, the latter with or without sub-headings, tables, illustrations, as the topic and treatment may require. The inclusion of a table or two, an illustration or two, does not automatically call for a list of tables and a list of illustrations; and for some papers a table of contents may have little value. These are matters, however, that must be left to the good sense of the writer, who should know best what arrangements are suitable for his particular piece of work.

The *order* of the following outline, regardless of the parts that may be omitted, should be observed.

a) *The front matter or preliminaries*, composed of
    (1) Title page (followed by a blank page).
    (2) Preface, including acknowledgments; or acknowledgments alone unless these appear as the final paragraph in the thesis.
    (3) Table of contents.
    (4) List of tables.
    (5) List of illustrations.
b) *The text*, composed of
    (1) Introduction.

---

[1] The term "paper" is used throughout this manual to refer alike to term papers, reports, theses, and dissertations except in matters relating specifically to one of them.

    (2) Half-title page.

    (3) Main body of the paper, usually consisting of well-defined divisions, such as chapters or their equivalents.[2]

c) *The reference matter*, composed of

    (1) Appendix.[2]

    (2) Bibliography.[2]

    (The order of these may be reversed.)

---

[2] If half-title pages are placed before groups of chapters, they should also be placed before the Appendix (or Appendixes) and the Bibliography.

II

Front Matter or Preliminaries

2. *Title page.*—Most universities and colleges have their own style of title page for theses and dissertations, and this should be followed exactly in matters of content and spacing. For term papers and reports, if a sample sheet is not provided, a title page might logically include the name of the university or college (usually centered at the top of the sheet), the exact title of the paper, the course, the date, and the name of the writer— all suitably capitalized, centered, and spaced upon the page.[1]

3. *Half-title page.*—Although not placed or numbered with the preliminaries, the half-title page may logically be mentioned here. It is necessary only for a paper in which the chapters are grouped into "parts." Consisting of a single page bearing the number and title of the part, it is placed immediately before the first of the chapters of which the part is composed.

If such half-title pages are needed, they should be placed also before the appendix (or appendixes) and the bibliography, the title "Appendix" or "Bibliography" replacing a part number and title.

4. *Preface or acknowledgments.*—Included in the preface (or

[1] All typing instructions, including the placement and capitalization of headings, margins, spacing, pagination, and the like, are given in Appendix I, "Typing the Paper" (pp. 127-39).

foreword) are such matters as the writer's reasons for making the study, its background, scope, and purpose, and acknowledgment of the aids afforded him in the process of the research and writing by institutions and persons. If the writer thinks he has nothing significant to say about the study that is not covered in the main body of the paper and wishes only to acknowledge the assistance of various sorts that he has received, he should entitle his remarks "Acknowledgments" instead of "Preface."[2]

5. *Table of contents.*—This sets forth the major divisions of the paper: the introduction, the chapters (or their equivalents, which need not be designated as chapters), with their numbers and titles, the appendix, and the bibliography, with their respective page numbers. The preliminaries are not usually included in the table of contents, but they may be, except for the contents itself. Subdivisions may or may not be included. (Instructions for the typing of the table of contents are on pp. 131-33, and three styles of contents are shown in the examples on pp. 152-54.)

6. *List of tables.*—This gives the table numbers with their individual headings and page numbers. (See instructions for typing, pp. 133-34, and sample in the Appendix, p. 155.)

7. *List of illustrations.*—If the illustrations consist of both plates and figures, the list may be divided under the subheadings "Plates" and "Figures," with individual numbers, titles, and page numbers shown for each kind. (Instructions for typing this list are on p. 134, and a sample is included in the Appendix, p. 155.)

2 Although the student would wish to acknowledge special assistance such as consultation on technical matters and aid in the securing of unusual equipment and source materials, he may with propriety omit an expression of formal thanks for the routine help given by an adviser or a thesis committee.

III

Text

8. *Introduction.*—The text ordinarily begins with an introduction, which may be Chapter I. If it is short, the writer may prefer to head it simply "Introduction," and reserve the more formal heading "Chapter" for the longer sections of which the main body of the paper is composed. But the Introduction, whether it is called Chapter I or not, is the first major division of the text, not the last of the preliminaries, as is sometimes supposed. Thus the first page of the Introduction is page 1 (Arabic numeral) of the paper.

9. *Chapters or their equivalents.*—The main body of the paper is usually divided into chapters, each chapter having a title and each beginning on a new page. For a short paper some writers prefer to omit the word "Chapter" and to use merely Roman numerals in sequence before the headings of the several main divisions of the paper. On the other hand, for a long paper some writers like to group related chapters into "parts," with or without individual titles (see sample, p. 153). Each part, then, is preceded by a half-title page indicating the chapters of which it is composed.

10. *Sections and subsections.*—In many papers the chapters or their equivalents are divided into sections, and sometimes further into one or more series of subsections, each preceded by a subtitle. The plan for the display of subtitles depends upon the

5

number of series of subsections to be shown. The style of heading with the greatest attention value must be given to the sections, and headings in a descending order of attention value to the subsections and sub-subsections. It is commonly agreed that centered headings have greater attention value than side headings and that underlined headings have greater attention value than those not underlined. Supposing, then, that five levels of subtitles were required, the following scheme would be appropriate:

a) Centered heading, underlined.

b) Centered heading, not underlined.

c) Side heading (that is, flush with the left margin), underlined.

d) Side heading, not underlined.

e) Paragraph heading (that is, a heading run into the paragraph, followed by a period and a dash), underlined.

If fewer than five levels are required, they might be selected in any suitable *descending order* as indicated in *a*) to *e*) above. (For additional information, see p. 135.)

11. *Titles in text.*—The same rules should be followed in text as in footnotes for the capitalization and underlining of certain titles and the "quoting" of others (see secs. 25, 26, 27, pp. 43-45.)

12. *Numbers.*—The general rule for ordinary text matter in which numbers appear in isolation is to spell out those under three digits and to use numerals for those of three digits or more.

Of the 210 families in the area studied, twenty-four had no children of elementary-school age.

Exceptions

The exceptions, however, are many.

a) In a group containing both numbers under and numbers over three digits, numerals should be used for all.

In the area studied, there are 186 such buildings, the smaller housing anywhere from 50 to 65 each, and the larger from 650 to over 1,000 each. One room may have as many as 8 occupants.

b) In a technical or a statistical discussion involving frequent numbers, use numerals for all.

The recommended daily dietary allowances for boys and girls 13 to 15 years of age; weight, 108 pounds; height, 64 inches; calls for 3,200 calories for boys and 2,600 for girls; protein allowance, 85 grams for boys and 80 for girls. . . .

c) For percentages, decimals, exact sums of money, and numbers combined with abbreviations (the last suitable only in scientific, technical, or statistical discussions), numerals should be used. "Per cent" should be spelled out.

With interest at 8 per cent, the monthly payment would amount to $12.88. This, he figured later, was exactly 2.425 times the amount he had hitherto saved monthly.

d) Street numbers and telephone numbers should never be spelled out.

e) Dates should be expressed in numerals except when the day of the month precedes the name of the month, or when the month is not given.

He was born on December 25, 1872. But his family always celebrated his birthday on the twenty-fourth.

f) Ordinals and fractions should be spelled out except when the fraction is part of a number of three digits or more.

twentieth century   one-tenth
Fifth Avenue   But: 124-1/2

g) The time of day should be spelled out except when A.M. or P.M. is used.

The meeting was called for eight o'clock.
The meeting was called for 8:00 P.M.

h) A sentence should never be started with a numeral, even

when there are numerals in the rest of the sentence. Either
spell out the first number or, better, recast the sentence.

Two hundred and fifty passengers escaped injury; 98 sustained
minor injuries, and 34 were so seriously hurt that they required
hospitalization; 5 were killed outright.

There were 250 passengers who escaped injury; 98 sustained minor
injuries. . . .

i) For reference to parts of a written work use numerals as
follows:

(1) lower-case Roman numerals (i, ii, iv, x, etc.) to indicate chapter, scene, canto, preliminary pages (preface, contents, etc.);

(2) capital Roman numerals (I, II, IV, X, etc.) to indicate volume, part, division, act (of a play), book,
plate;

(3) Arabic numerals to indicate pages other than preliminaries; all divisions of classical works; column, line,
table, figure, and possibly other divisions.

13. *Enumerations:*

a) *Run on in text.*—Numbers and letters used to enumerate
items in text stand out better when set in parentheses (either
single or double) than when followed by periods.

The reasons for his resignation were three: (1) advanced age,
(2) failing health, (3) a desire to travel.

b) *Beginning a new line or paragraph.*—But when numbered
items in an enumeration without subdivisions begin each
on a new line, Arabic numerals followed by periods should
ordinarily be used. The periods should always be aligned.

8. Purchase of supplies.
9. Operation of physical plant.
10. Reduction in cost of collecting school funds.

c) *In outline form.*—For an outline or other enumeration

having several subdivisions, the following scheme of notation and indention should be used:

```
 I. Wars of the Nineteenth Century
    A. United States
       1. Civil War, 1861-65
          a) Causes
             (1) Slavery
                (a) Compromise
                    i) Missouri Compromise
                   ii) Compromise of 1850

II. Under the head of . . .
    A. Under the head of . . .
       1. Under the head of . . .
             ETC.
```

14. *Spelling.*—In general, spelling (as well as syllabication) should accord with the best American usage, and it must be consistent, except, of course, in quotations. The authority should be the latest edition of *Webster's New International Dictionary*. For the spelling of personal names, reference should be made to *Webster's Biographical Dictionary*, and for geographical names, to *Webster's Geographical Dictionary*.

a) *Plural of proper nouns:*

   (1) Form the plural of proper nouns by adding *s*, except for nouns ending with a sibilant not followed by *e*.

the Audleys	the Baylors	the McLeods
the Andersons	the Costellos	the Pettees
		the Boyces

   (2) Form the plural of proper nouns ending in a sibilant, other than those ending in a sibilant and *e*, by adding *es*.

the Rosses	the Diazes	the Markses
the Stevenses	the Foxes	But: the Boyces

b) *Possessive of proper nouns:*

   (1) Form the possessive singular of one-syllable proper nouns ending in *s* or another sibilant and *e*, by adding an apostrophe and *s*.

```
Wells's novels        Marx's theories        Joyce's boat
Keats's poems         Jones's house
```

(2) Form the possessive singular of proper nouns of *more than one syllable* that end in *s* or another sibilant by adding an apostrophe only, except that for nouns ending with a sibilant and *e*, and those ending with a *silent z*, add an apostrophe and *s*.

```
Praxiteles' sculpture    But: Horace's odes
Jeffers' poems                Clarice's grades
Berlioz' music                Agassiz's research
```

(3) Form the possessive plural of proper nouns by adding an apostrophe to the accepted form of the plural of the noun (see *a*, 1 and 2, above).

```
the Rosses' boat         the Costellos' house
the Stevenses' camp      the Andersons' car
the McLeods' son         the Joyces' dog
```

c) *Plural and possessive of prepositional-phrase compounds.* —Note that although the plural of such compounds is written, for example:

```
brothers-in-law      commanders-in-chief      men-of-war
```

the possessive case is:

```
brother-in-law's     commander-in-chief's     man-of-war's
```

15. *Division of words and other separations at ends of lines.*—In general, divide words according to syllabication as shown in *Webster's Dictionary*. There, the syllables are separated by a heavy dot, except that following the accented syllable the accent mark serves the dual purpose of indicating syllabication as well as stress in pronunciation: *syl·lab·i·ca′tion.*

Some exceptions to the general rule and some peculiarities of syllabication are illustrated in the following:

a) *Never* make a one-letter division.

```
Wrong: u-nite    a-mong    e-nough    man-y
```

b) *Never* carry over *-ed* if the word is pronounced as one syllable.

<u>Wrong</u>: aim-ed   climb-ed   help-ed   pass-ed

c) *Never* divide the final syllables *-able* and *-ible*.

<u>Wrong</u>: inevita-ble   permissi-ble   allowa-ble
<u>Right</u>: inevit-able   permiss-ible   allow-able

d) *Never* divide the following suffixes:

-cial   -cion   -tion   -geous
-sial   -gion   -ceous   -gious
-tial   -sion   -cious   -tious

e) *Never* divide a proper *name* unless the correct division has first been learned by consulting a biographical dictionary, or unless it is a name of which the correct division is obvious.

Wash-ing-ton   Dear-born   Jef-fer-son   Went-worth

f) Avoid two-letter divisions.

<u>Not</u>: mon-ey   ris-en   loss-es   pray-er   stat-ed

g) Avoid divisions of hyphenated words.

<u>Not</u>: court-mar-tial   pres-i-dent-elect   un-Chris-tian

h) The final syllable *-ing* may always be carried over except when the ending consonant of the parent word is doubled before *-ing*.

will-ing   <u>But</u>: win-ning
carry-ing   control-ling
connect-ing   scar-ring

i) Note that in some words whose ending-consonant sounds belong to a syllable with a silent vowel, such consonants become part of the added syllable *-ing* or *-ed*.

han-dling   bris-tling   chuck-ling   ruf-fling   twin-kling
han-dled   bris-tled   chuck-led   ruf-fled   twin-kled

j) *Never* divide (i.e., put in different lines) the initials of a name or the first name and the initial; the month and the day; capital letters as abbreviations for the names of any of the following: countries and states (U.S., N.Y.), organizations (YMCA, NATO), publications and editions (OED, R.S.V.), radio and television stations (KFRC, KQED; but two *sets* of initials separated by a hyphen, e.g., KRON-FM, may be divided after the hyphen), academic titles (M.D., B.A., Ph.D.); a numeral, letter, or symbol from the element it designates; or any such combinations as the following: £6 4s. 6d, 400 B.C., 6:00 P.M.

k) *Never* end a line with an opening quotation mark, or an opening parenthesis, or an opening bracket; and *never* begin a line with a final quotation mark, or a final parenthesis, or a final bracket, or with any mark of punctuation except an opening quotation mark, or an opening parenthesis, or an opening bracket.

m) For rules on the division of words in foreign languages, the *Manual of Style* should be consulted. As in English, there are divisions that are forbidden and others to be avoided, and neither is shown in general dictionaries.

16. *Abbreviations.*—Generally speaking, aside from the exceptions noted below, abbreviations should not be used in *the text*.

a) Spell out all the following: names of states, counties, provinces, and so on; days of the week and months; expressions of dimension, distance, measure, and weight; the words "page," "section," "book," "volume," "chapter," "column," "line," "figure," "plate," and so on; the words "street," "avenue," "terrace," and so on; the parts of geographic names (e.g., North Carolina, Fort Wayne, Mount Whitney, *but* St. Louis; the words "company," "brother," "associate," "incorporated," "and" (in place of the ampersand [&]), even when forming part of the name of a commercial firm; titles preceding personal names (e.g., Professor Lewis, General Lee, Senator Clark).

Exceptions

b) Use the following abbreviations before names: Mr., Messrs., Mrs. (and their foreign equivalents, such as the French M., MM., Mme, Mlle), Dr., St. (for Saint, not Street), Ste., Rev., and Hon.[1]

c) When placed after the names, abbreviate Sr., Jr., and Esq., and all academic degrees, B.A., M.S., Ph.D., LL.D.

d) When they are preceded by the hour, abbreviate A.M. and P.M.

e) When they are used with dates, abbreviate B.C. and A.D.

f) In exact references to passages of Scripture, abbreviate the books of the Bible, the Apocrypha, and the Apocalyptic, using standard abbreviations such as those in *A Manual of Style*, or in such a commentary as *The Interpreter's Bible*, or in the Bible itself.

   The various versions of the Bible are commonly referred to by their abbreviations: Vulg., D.V., R.S.V., E.R.V.

g) Many governmental divisions, as well as committees, agencies, associations, unions, and the like, are so well known by their abbreviations that these may be safely used without further identification. But if the organization is not well known, spell out the name the first time it occurs and place after it in parentheses the abbreviation that will be used thereafter. Notice that all such abbreviations omit space and periods between them: FHA, CIA, FBI, UNESCO, NATO, OAS, YMCA, IOOF, CIO, AFL.

h) Radio and television stations are referred to by their abbreviations in the same style as that used for governmental agencies: KRON-FM, WGN-TV, WMAQ, KQED. But

---

[1] *Never* use Rev. or Hon. (or Reverend or Honorable) before a surname alone. Follow it either with the forename or the initials or the appropriate title: Rev. J. Cyril Stevens, or the Reverend J. Cyril Stevens, or Rev. Dr. Stevens, or Rev. Mr. Stevens, or simply Mr. Stevens. When "the" *precedes either* Reverend or Honorable, the latter should be spelled out.

the abbreviations of broadcasting companies place periods, without space, after the letters: "N.B.C.," "C.B.S.," "A.B.C.," "B.B.C."

i) Although abbreviations other than the foregoing should not be used in text, they not only are allowable but are preferable in lists and tables and, in some instances, in footnotes. Also, exceptions are made for papers in scientific fields (see chap. ix).

17. *Foreign words and phrases.*—Underline foreign words and phrases in English text.

> Clearly, this . . . leads to the idea of <u>Ubermensch</u> and also to the theory of the <u>acte gratuit</u> and surrealism.

Exceptions

a) The words in a quotation entirely in a foreign language are not normally underlined. In the following sentence, the words *le pragmatisme* are properly underlined, and the quotation, entirely in French, is properly not underlined:

> The confusion of <u>le pragmatisme</u> is traced to the supposed failure to distinguish "les propriétés de la valeur en général" from the incidental.

But in the following French quotation, some words are properly underlined because they are used by the writer as examples:

> ... quand j'ai dû analyser le style de Wright ... j'ai été frappé par l'emploi ironique de ses conjonctions causales (<u>à cause</u>, <u>parce que</u>, etc.).

And in the following sentences, French words are both "quoted" and underlined because of the special way in which they are used:

> The realist novelist is seen by the author as essentially an unmasker, a "<u>dénonciateur</u>."

> This is what the French call "<u>la fortune</u>."

b) Foreign titles preceding proper names, and foreign names of persons, places, institutions, and the like, are not underlined.

Père Grou	the Teatro Real	the German
M. Jacquet, Ministre	the Puerta del	Bundestag
de Travaux	Sol	the Quai d'Orsay
the Académie	the Vienna	the Arc de
Française	Staatsoper	Triomphe

c) Foreign words which by continued use in English have become Anglicized are not underlined. Some of the more common are listed below (consult *Webster's Dictionary* and *A Manual of Style* for others). Notice that some have dropped the accent marks proper to their native forms. The greater number, however, retain the marks, and they must be inserted by hand, in permanent black ink, unless your typewriter is equipped with them. It is *never permissible* to substitute an apostrophe for the grave or for the acute accent mark.

a posteriori	coup de grâce	per cent
a priori	debris	per se
ad hoc	denouement	pro rata
ad infinitum	de rigueur	rapport
ante bellum	dilettante	rapprochement
apropos	entree	recherché
attaché	entrepreneur	regime
beau ideal	ex officio	résumé
bête noire	exposé	role
blitzkrieg	genre	status quo
bona fide	habeas corpus	subpoena
bourgeoisie	laissez faire	tête-à-tête
carte blanche	milieu	versus
chargé d'affaires	mores	via
cliché	naïveté	vice versa
communiqué	par excellence	vis-à-vis
contretemps	per annum	visa
coup d'état	per capita	Weltanschauung

IV

Quotations

18. In general, quotations should correspond exactly with the originals in wording, spelling, capitalization, and punctuation. Exceptions to the general rule are discussed under "Ellipses," "Interpolations," and "Italics" (pp. 20-25).

   a) Prose.—Short direct prose quotations should be incorporated into the text of the paper and enclosed in double quotation marks. But, in general, a prose quotation of two or more sentences which *at the same time* runs to four or more typewritten lines should be set off from the text in single spacing and indented in its entirety four spaces from the left marginal line, with no quotation marks at beginning and end. Exceptions to this rule are allowable when for purposes of emphasis or of comparison it is desirable to single-space and indent quotations less than four typewriten lines in length. Paragraph indention in the original text should be indicated by an eight-space indention from the left marginal line, as for a paragraph in the text of the paper. (See sample page, p. 157.) Double-space between the text and the indented, single-spaced quotation, but single-space between the paragraphs of the quotation, except when passages are quoted from different works of the same author or from different authors, in which cases double-space between the separate passages.

   b) Poetry.—Quotations of poetry two or more lines in length should be set off from the text in single spacing. Use no quotation marks at beginning and end, except when citing from different works of the same author or from different authors. In general, the indention should be determined by centering the longest line, but if this is disproportionately long, the indention should be set by an average of the long lines. This is to say that the whole quoted section should appear to be centered upon the page. Verses of the same poem as well as those of different poems are separated with double spacing.

Upon occasion, it is suitable to insert two lines of verse directly into text—as, for example, in a critical examination of a poem. In such case, quotation marks are used and the lines separated by a virgule (/).

```
        In the valley the mariners find life's purpose reduced
to the simple naturalistic proposition, "All things have rest,
and ripen toward the grave / In silence, ripen, fall, and
cease."
```

c) *Mottoes.*—When used at the heads of chapters, mottoes (or epigraphs) are given the same indention as paragraphs and are not enclosed in quotation marks. The source, preceded by a dash (--), is placed below the motto and is aligned to end with it.

```
    A storm of mosquitoes may create a noise like thunder.
                                        --Old Chinese saying
```

d) *Quotations in footnotes.*—Whether run on in the body of a footnote or indented and set off from it, all quoted matter in footnotes is enclosed in quotation marks.

e) *Quotation marks.*—Primary quotations—other than those long quotations that are single-spaced and indented, as described in sections *a* and *b*, above—require double quotation marks to be placed at beginning and end. Thus, if double quotation marks appear in the original of the part quoted, those marks must be changed to single. On the other hand, in a single-spaced, indented quotation, where the marks are omitted at beginning and end, the quotation marks appearing within the original matter are retained.

(1) For a primary quotation, whether it consists of a single word, numeral, or letter, or of several words, double quotation marks are used.

    Twenty-one papers have been prepared under the captions
"Background," "Relation to Card Catalogs," "Techniques,"
"Standards," "Applications."

    The enumeration may be either numbered "1," "2," "3,"
etc., or lettered "a," "b," "c," etc.

(2) For a quotation within a quotation, single quotation marks are used; if within that quotation is another, double marks are again used; if yet another, single marks, and so on.

    The chairman reported as follows: "The mayor's repre-
sentative has replied: 'I am authorized by the Chamber of Commerce to make this offer, their provision stating, "The jobs
shall be made available provided that the committee guarantee
all the means for receiving applications." That guarantee has
been made, and the procedure outlined.'"

(3) In quoting a letter, opening quotation marks are placed at the beginning of each element of the address, of the salutation, of each paragraph, of the complimentary close, and of the signature. Closing quotation marks appear only at the end of the complete letter, that is, following the signature.[1]

---

[1] The use of quotation marks as set forth here and in sections 4 and 5 below does not reverse the rule given in section 18, *a*, which calls for the indention and single-spacing of long quotations and the omission of quotation marks at beginning and end. But because the writer of the paper may very well employ examples of his own and single-space and indent them—either for appearance or emphasis, or for both—and also cite similar materials taken from other writers, it is advisable for clarification that in the latter cases the quoted materials be indicated as such by enclosing them in quotation marks.

```
                                  "Baltimore, Maryland
                                  "June 1, 1965
"The University of Chicago
"Chicago, Illinois
"Gentlemen:
"Will you kindly let me have the following information
concerning . . .

                                  "Very truly yours,
                                  "Clyde L. Brown"
```

(4) Similarly, in an outline a quotation mark is placed before each unit and at the end of only the last.

```
Their outline for the third-year course is as follows:
"III. Predicate-element concept
    "A. Verb
        "1. Forms and uses of verb 'to be'
        "2. Tense
            "a) Present perfect
            "b) Past perfect"
```

(5) In a quotation that includes headings and/or subheadings, a quotation mark is placed before each heading and subheading as well as before each paragraph, with the closing quotation mark coming only at the end of the whole quotation.

```
                        "CHAPTER I


            "THE DEVELOPMENT OF A RACE RELATIONS

                    ACTION STRUCTURE


            "Race Relations in the British Isles
                    1700 to World War I

        "A small Negro population was living in London by 1700,
and some have estimated that by 1770 there were between 14,000
and 20,000 Negroes residing in greater London. . . .
. . . . . . . . . . . . . . . . . . . . . . . . . . . . . .
        "During the same period there were about 10,000
Irish, . . . "
```

f) *Punctuation next to the closing quotation mark.*—Periods and commas should always be placed inside quotation marks (even when the quotation marks enclose only one letter or figure); semicolons and colons, outside. Question marks and exclamation marks should be placed outside the quotation marks unless the question or the exclamation occurs within the wording of the quotation.

> Does he precisely show "evil leading somehow to good"?

> One may well ask: "Is it really necessary to lose the world in order to find ourselves?"

> The cries of "Long live the King!" echoed down the broad avenues.

Exceptions

g) *Ellipses.*—An omission within a quoted sentence is shown by three spaced periods (i.e., a space before each period and after the last).

> In conclusion he stated: "What we require to be taught . . . is to be our own teachers."

(1) If there is punctuation immediately before the ellipsis, the mark is placed next to the word it follows in the quotation. Since ellipsis marks replace words in a quotation, notice that they are always put inside the quotation marks.

> "We are fighting . . . for the holy cause of Slavdom, . . . for freedom, . . . for the Orthodox cross. . . ."

(2) If there is a punctuation mark immediately preceding the word following the ellipsis, the mark comes after the ellipsis.

> "All this is not exactly in S's tradition . . . , and not in your style at the start of the war."

(3) When an ellipsis follows a complete sentence, a terminal period (or another mark of terminal punctuation) is placed at the end of the sentence, with three ellipsis marks following.

"When a nation is clearly in the wrong, it ought not to
be too proud to say so. . . . I have not been enunciating principles which we do not apply in our own case."

(4) Views differ with respect to the use of ellipsis marks at the beginning and end of quotations consisting of partial sentences not ending with terminal punctuation.

It has been pointed out that in wording, spelling, and punctuation, quotations must be exactly reproduced. But following long-established practice, some writers change the capitalization of the first word of a quotation in accordance with the following rule. If the text matter introducing the quotation ends either with terminal punctuation or with a colon, the first word is capitalized even though it may be uncapitalized in the original; but if the quotation is closely joined grammatically to the writer's introductory words, the first word of the quotation is begun with a small letter, although it may be capitalized in the original.

The following day Sand reported: "With Pebble soliciting members on the side, it was imperative that the meeting be
no longer delayed." [In the original, "With" occurs within a
sentence and is therefore uncapitalized.]

The Act provided that "the General Counsel of the Board
shall exercise general supervision." [In the original, "the"
is the first word of the sentence and is therefore capitalized.]

Other writers, out of regard both for the integrity of the original and ease in locating quotations, hold out for ellipsis marks to be placed before the first word when it occurs within a sentence and is therefore uncapitalized in the original. They would write unhesitatingly:

The following day Sand reported: " . . . with Pebble
soliciting members . . . "

There is similar difference of opinion regarding the use of ellipsis marks at the end of quotations. Some

writers maintain that if the quoted matter is grammatically complete, terminal punctuation, followed
immediately by the closing quotation mark, is appropriate, even though the original shows a weaker mark
at the end of the quotation.

```
     "Part of the historical problem concerns the state of
affairs in Spain in the period, and part concerns the state of
affairs in the Spanish Netherlands." [In the original, a semi-
colon follows "Netherlands."]
```

The same considerations that prompt some writers
to insert ellipsis marks at the beginning of quotations
dictate their use at the end following a weak mark of
punctuation.

```
     "Part of the historical problem concerns the state of
affairs in Spain in the period, and part concerns the state of
affairs in the Spanish Netherlands; . . . "
```

One scheme should be followed consistently
throughout the paper, both for quotations run on in
text and those that are indented and single-spaced.

(5) Incomplete quoted expressions employed in such a
sentence as the following require ellipsis marks before
the last quotation mark in each case.

```
The summary should be introduced by an appropriate transitional
expression such as, "In summary . . . ," "On the whole . . . ,"
"As has been said. . . . "
```

(6) In a single-spaced, indented quotation, the omission
of a paragraph or more is indicated by a full line of
ellipsis marks. The full line of marks, however, does
not cover the omission (if any) of the last part of the
paragraph preceding, which must have its own appropriate marks, as shown below:

```
  1. The paper must include a discussion of the moral bases and
     social effects of the kind of ownership which you favor or
     wish to attack. . . .
     . . . . . . . . . . . . . . . . . . . . . . . . . . . . . . . .
  4. In form, the paper must be an argument; . . .
     . . . . . . . . . . . . . . . . . . . . . . . . . . . . . . . .
```

In such a quotation as the foregoing, a full line of
ellipsis marks at the end is used to indicate that the
outline continues beyond the point quoted. In a quoted
passage of straight prose, such a full line of ellipsis
marks is rarely needed at the end. If, however, the
concluding part of a paragraph is omitted and the paragraph following it is quoted, that omission should be
appropriately indicated by three ellipsis marks plus
a punctuation mark.

(7) Similarly, in a verse quotation the omission of a full
line, or more than one full line, is indicated by a single
line of ellipsis marks. Note that the full line of ellipsis
marks, whether in a prose or in a verse quotation,
does not extend beyond the longest type line of the
quotation.

```
Dear is the memory of our wedded lives,
And dear the last embraces of our wives.
. . . . . . . . . . . . . . . . . . . . . .
Our sons inherit us: our looks are strange:
And we should come like ghosts to trouble joy.
```

(8) Now the question may be asked: How are such long
omissions (as those just mentioned) indicated in quotations that are run on in text? Not, indeed, by a complete line of ellipsis marks, but rather by separate
quotations such as those shown in the example under
(5) above. Nor, according to a mistaken notion, do the
ellipsis marks appear *between* the quotations. It must
be remembered that since ellipsis marks indicate omissions *within* quotations, they should always be placed
within the quotation marks (although the quotation
marks do not appear in indented, single-spaced quotations).

<u>Right</u>: "The project underwent thorough evaluation and was intro-
duced to guide the hospital in future planning; . . . "
"Modification of admission policies was worked out;
. . . " "The research added a new dimension."

<u>Wrong</u>: "The project underwent thorough evaluation and was intro-
duced to guide the hospital in future planning;" . . .
"Modification of admission policies was worked out;"
. . . "The research added a new dimension."

(9) Omissions in Latin and in German text employ ellipsis marks as in English.

(10) In French and Spanish text, omissions within a sentence are indicated by three periods without space between, but with a space before the first mark and one after the third mark. Any punctuation mark preceding the ellipsis is placed immediately next to the word it follows.

"Ma lettre d'audience? ... Pourquoi faire? ... Je suis, certes,
assez bon ami du roi ... mais j'ai besoin qu'on m'annonce. ...
Je ne m'annoncerai pas bien moi-même! ... "

(11) In Italian text, any omission is indicated by four unspaced periods followed by a space. Any mark of punctuation immediately preceding the omission replaces the first period.

"Dio mio!... Non c'è voce umana che muova il tuo cuore
feroce?... "

h) *Interpolations.*—At times the writer finds it advisable to insert into a quotation a word or more of explanation, clarification, or correction. All such interpolations must be placed between square brackets []. Parenthesis may *not* be substituted; if the typewriter has no brackets, they must be inserted in the copy by hand, in permanent black ink.

To assure the reader that the faulty logic, error in fact, incorrect word, incorrect spelling, or the like, is in the original, the Latin word *sic* ("so"; always underlined) may be placed after the error.

"When the fog lifted, they were delighted to see that the country was heavily timbered and emmence [sic] numbers of fowl flying in every direction."

The use of *sic* should not be overdone. Quotations from a work of the sixteenth century, for example, or from obviously archaic or illiterate writing, should not be strewn with *sic*'s.

Interpolations made for the purposes of correction and clarification are illustrated in the following:

"But since these masters [Picasso, Braque, Matisse] appeared to be throwing away, rebelling against academic training, art teaching has itself been discredited."

"The recipient of the Nobel Peace Award for 1961 [1960] was Albert John Luthuli."

i) *Italics.*—Words that are not italicized in the original may be italicized (underlined) for emphasis desired by the writer of the paper. This change may be indicated to the reader in one of three ways.

(1) By a notation enclosed in square brackets placed immediately after the underlined words, as in the following:

"This man described to me another large river beyond the Rocky Mountains, the southern branch [italics mine] of which he directed me to take."

(2) By a parenthetical note following the quotation.

"This man described to me another large river beyond the Rocky Mountains, the southern branch of which he directed me to take." (Italics mine.)

(3) By a footnote. Either a footnote or the scheme mentioned in (2) above is preferable when italics have been added at two or more points in a quotation.

V

Footnotes

19. *Their use.*—Footnotes have four main uses: (*a*) to cite the authority for statements in text—specific facts or opinions as well as exact quotations;[1] (*b*) to make incidental comments upon, to amplify or to qualify textual discussion—in short, to provide a place for material which the writer thinks it worthwhile to include but which he feels would disrupt the flow of thought if introduced into the text; (*c*) to make cross-references; (*d*) to make acknowledgments. Footnotes, then, are of two kinds, *reference* (*a* and *c* above), and *content* (*b* and *d* above). A content footnote may also include one or more references, as will be seen in the examples (sec. 45, pp. 64-65). Interpretations and examples of footnote form are given in the following pages.

20. *Footnote numbers.*—The place in text at which a footnote is introduced, whether of the reference or of the content type, should be marked with an Arabic numeral. Place the numeral slightly above the line (but never a full space above), and do not put a period after it or embellish it with parentheses, brackets, or slashes. The numeral follows a punctuation mark, if any, except

---

[1] Such authority is usually a written source, published or unpublished. When a general rather than a specific term must be used to refer to such a source, it is called in this manual a "work"; or, where its form needs to be more clearly indicated, a "whole work" or a "whole published work" to refer to a separate publication, and a "part" or a "component part" to refer to some division of the whole.

for the dash, which it precedes. The footnote number should follow the passage to which it refers. If the passage is an exact quotation, the footnote number comes at the end of the quotation, not after the author's name or at the end of the textual matter introducing the quotation.

Footnote numbers should follow each other in numerical order on the page. They may begin with "l" (a small "l," not a capital "I," is used for the Arabic numeral one) on each page, or with "l" at the beginning of each chapter, or they may run in one series through the entire paper. There are possible complications in using the last two schemes, however, since if it was found that a note had been omitted, or that one should be deleted, it would be necessary to renumber the footnotes from the point of the desired change to the end of the chapter or of the paper. The insertion of a note numbered, for example, "la" is not permissible, and the omission of a number likewise is not permissible.

21. *Placement of footnotes.*—Footnotes should be arranged in numerical order at the foot of the page, and all those to which references are made in the text must appear on the same page as the references.

Reduction in the number of reference numbers in the text improves the appearance of the page and saves space in the footnote area as well as in typing time. Consider the spotty effect and the waste space resulting from a line or a column of *ibid.*'s. With careful planning, the number of footnotes and their bulk as well can often be considerably reduced without curtailing scholarly responsibilities. Three ways may be mentioned.

a) In a *single* paragraph containing several quotations from one work of the same author, a reference number following the last quotation would permit all the quotations to be cited in one footnote.

b) Instead of four reference numbers in such a sentence as the following: "Assertions about the value of this legislation were made by Ames,[1] Brett,[2] Connor,[3] and Frank,[4]" one number placed after the last name would allow all four citations to be made in one footnote. The sentence in the text would read, "Assertions about the value of this legislation were made by Ames, Brett, Connor, and Frank.[1]" The footnote would be:

[1]Lumsden B. Ames, *Title of work* (facts of publication if the work has not been previously cited), p. 00; Frank P. Brett, information corresponding to that given for Ames; Reginald J. Connor, information corresponding to that given for Ames; Azariah D. Frank, information corresponding to that given for Ames.

c) Unless they are very short and uncomplicated, tables, outlines, lists, letters, and the like that are not immediately relevant to the text may be placed in an appendix at the back of the book rather than in footnotes. So placed, a simple note takes care of the reference in the text.

[1]The member banks and their contributions are listed in Appendix II.

Specific directions for the typing of footnotes and for their correct placement on the page are given in Appendix I (pp. 137-39).

REFERENCE FOOTNOTES: BASIC FORMS
FIRST, FULL REFERENCES

22. *Basic style.*—The first time a work is mentioned in a footnote,[1] the entry should be in complete form; that is, it should include not only the author's full name, the title, and the volume and/or page number, but it should give the facts of publication as well.

[1] Sample footnote references with corresponding bibliographic entries are shown in chapter vii, pp. 73-81.

The last may be omitted, however, provided that the work is included in the bibliography. Once a work has been cited in full, subsequent references to it may be in abbreviated form. These forms are fully discussed and illustrated on pages 59-64.

With some exceptions, such as references to legal, classical, and biblical works, to certain classes of public documents, and to references in scientific papers—all discussed hereinafter—footnotes citing a published work the first time are given in the sequence indicated below. Although not every footnote entry will include all the items of information mentioned, the order should be maintained regardless of the items omitted.

For a book, the source of the information, except the page number(s), should be the title page; for a periodical, it should be the cover and the article itself.

a) *For a book:*
    (1) Name of author(s) (pp. 30-31).[1]
    (2) Title of book (p. 32).
    (3) Name of editor or translator, if any (p. 33).
    (4) Name of series in which the book appears, if any, and volume or number in the series (pp. 34-35).
    (5) Facts of publication, consisting of
        (a) Total number of volumes, if relevant (p. 36).
        (b) Number of edition, if other than the first (p. 36).
        (c) Place of publication (pp. 36-37).
        (d) Name of publishing agency (pp. 37-39).
        (e) Date of publication (pp. 39-40).
    (6) Volume number, if necessary (pp. 40-41).
    (7) Page number(s) (p. 42).

b) *For an article in a periodical:*
    (1) Same as (1) above (pp. 30-31).
    (2) Title of article (p. 32).
    (3) Name of periodical (p. 32).

---

[1] The pages noted in parentheses following each item refer to the detailed discussion.

(4) Volume (and number, if any), of periodical (pp. 40-41).

(5) Date of volume or issue (p. 41).

(6) Page number(s) (p. 42).

c) Under their separate heads, the items of information listed in *a* and *b* above will now be discussed in detail.

(1) *Name of author.*—Give the author's name in normal order—Robert John Blank—and follow it with a comma. Give the first name(s), not initials only, except for well-known authors who habitually use only the initials of their first names (e.g., D. H. Lawrence, T. S. Eliot, W. B. Yeats, P. G. Wodehouse, J. B. S. Haldane). For an author whose first names appear in some of the works cited and initials only in others, the footnote references to the latter should write the name, for example, H[enry] R[obert] Anderson. But for the works in which the first names are spelled out, the references should give the name as Henry Robert Anderson.

If the title page (or the byline of an article) bears a pseudonym known to be that of a certain author, the real name, placed between brackets, follows the pseudonym (see example *g*, p. 74). Such familiar pseudonyms as Anatole France, George Eliot, and Mark Twain should be excepted, however.

If a pseudonym is indicated as such on the title page, the abbreviation "pseud." is enclosed in parentheses and placed after the name—Helen Delay (pseud.).

If pseudonymity is not indicated on the title page but it is nevertheless an established fact, the abbreviation "pseud." may be placed in brackets after the name—Helen Delay [pseud.].

If the title page mentions no author, or if it designates the work as anonymous, and the authorship has been definitely established, the author's name may be enclosed in brackets and placed before the title— [Henry K. Black].

For a work by more than one author, the full names are set down in normal order, separated by commas and the last comma followed by "and" ("and" without comma between two names). If a work has more than three authors, it is usual to cite for the footnote (but not for the bibliography) only the name of the first author mentioned on the title page and to follow it either with "*et al.*" (*et alii*) or with the English equivalent, "and others" (see example, p. 74). Use only *one* style throughout the paper, and if you choose to employ "*et al.*" or "and others," cite before it only the name of the first author.

For co-authors with the same surname, cite each name in full in the first reference—Sidney Webb and Beatrice Webb, not Sidney and Beatrice Webb. In later references write Webb and Webb, not the Webbs.

Even though title pages may include after authors' names such titles as doctor, professor, president, or academic degrees or official positions held by the authors, all such are omitted except in rare instances of their having special significance for the subject discussed.

The "author" may be a corporate body—a country, state, city, legislative body, institution, society, business firm, or the like (see p. 75).

Some works—compilations for the most part—are produced by compilers or editors rather than authors (see example, p. 75).

When a work does not bear the name of an author, editor, or compiler, the footnote references begin with the title of the work, not (except in very rare instances) with "Anonymous."

(2) *Title of the work.*—Enter the title of a book as it appears on the title page. Enter the title of an article in a periodical as it appears at the head of the article, and follow with the name of the periodical, placing a comma between them. Adhere to the peculiarities of spelling and to the punctuation within the titles, but capitalize in conformance with the scheme adopted for the paper as a whole (see pp. 44-45).

Underline the title of a whole published work—that is, underline the title of a book and the name of a periodical; quote (i.e., place between quotation marks) the title of an article in a periodical. Place a comma after the title of a book, after the title of an article, and after the name of a periodical, unless in the title it is followed immediately by parentheses enclosing the facts of publication, when the comma is placed after the closing parenthesis.

Arthur C. Kirsch, <u>Dryden's Heroic Drama</u> (Princeton, N.J.: Princeton University Press, 1964), p. 15.

Samuel M. Thompson, "The Authority of Law," <u>Ethics</u>, LXXV (October, 1964), 16-24.

Since display headings, both on title pages and at the heads of articles, frequently set a title in two or more lines and since punctuation is commonly omitted at the ends of display headings, it is frequently necessary to add marks of punctuation to a title. This occurs most often in titles composed of a main title and a subtitle. In the following, for example, *The Early Growth of Logic in the Child: Classification and Seriation,* the subtitle, *Classification and Seriation,* appears on a separate line and there is no punctuation following *Child.* Copied without change from the title page, the title looks like this:

Wrong: <u>The Early Growth of Logic in the Child Classification and Seriation</u>.

Adding a colon after *Child* clarifies the meaning.

Right: <u>The Early Growth of Logic in the Child: Classification and Seriation</u>.

(3) *Names of editors, compilers, translators.*—If the title page indicates in addition to the name of an author that of an editor, compiler, or translator, that name is placed after the title, the name being preceded by "ed." or "comp." or "trans.," as is appropriate. (A work may have both an editor and a translator as well as an author.)

Helmut Thielicke, <u>Man in God's World</u>, trans. and ed. by John W. Doberstein (New York and Evanston: Harper & Row, 1963), p. 43.

Similar in style is the entry of a work in which the author's name is contained in the title. In such case the separate entry of the author's name is omitted.

<u>The Works of Shakespear</u>, ed. by Alexander Pope (6 vols.; London: Printed for Jacob Tonson in the Strand, 1723-25), II, 38.

Although the foregoing is the style of reference most commonly used for such a work, in a paper dealing with the work of Alexander Pope, his name as editor might well precede the title.

Alexander Pope, ed., <u>The Works of Shakespear</u> (6 vols.; London: Printed for Jacob Tonson in the Strand, 1723-25), II, 38.

(4) *Name of author of preface, foreword, or introduction.*—When a book carries a preface, a foreword, or an introduction written by a distinguished person, its inclusion with the author's name is often indicated on the title page. The reference to such a book takes the following form.

Dag Hammarskjöld, <u>Markings</u>, with a Foreword by W. H.
Auden (New York: Alfred A. Knopf, Inc., 1964).

(5) *Name of series.*—Books and pamphlets are often
published as parts of a named series (e.g., Oxford
Standard Authors, Social Work Curriculum Study,
Studies in East European History). But first it is
necessary to note the difference between a series, a
multivolume work, and a periodical, since each has its
particular style of reference. Their main difference is
in plan of publication.

A multivolume work is one within limits more or less
clearly defined before publication. It consists, or will
consist, of a number of volumes related to the same
subject. All the volumes may be the work of one author
and all bear the same title (n. 1), or each a different
title (n. 2), or they may be by different authors and
bear different titles. In the last case, there is an editor—
perhaps more than one—of the complete work, which
carries an over-all title (n. 3).

[1]Paul Tillich, <u>Systematic Theology</u> (3 vols.; Chicago:
University of Chicago Press, 1951-53), II, 48.

[2]Gerald E. Bentley, <u>The Jacobean and Caroline Stage</u>,
Vols. I-II: <u>Dramatic Companies and Players</u>; Vols. III-V: <u>Plays
and Playwrights</u> (Oxford: Clarendon Press, 1941-56).

[3]Gordon N. Ray, gen. ed., <u>An Introduction to Literature</u>,
Vol. I: <u>Reading the Short Story</u>, by H. Barrows; Vol. II: <u>The
Nature of Drama</u>, by H. Hefner; Vol. III: <u>How Does a Poem Mean</u>,
by J. Ciardi; Vol. IV: <u>The Character of Prose</u>, by W. Douglas
(4 vols.; Boston: Houghton Mifflin Company, 1959).

A series is an ongoing project, the purpose of which
is the publication from time to time of books or
pamphlets by different writers on topics ranging often
rather widely over a specific field, or discipline, or area
of interest. Named series are sponsored by publishers,

institutions, governmental agencies, societies, commercial and industrial firms, and so on. Ordinarily each work bears a number in the series. The name of the series follows the title of the individual work. The accepted style of capitalization is used, but the name is not underlined or quoted.

Maximilien E. Novak, Defoe and the Nature of Man, Oxford English Monographs (London: Oxford University Press, 1963), p. 45.

National Industrial Conference Board, Research and Development, Studies in Business Economics, No. 82 (New York: National Industrial Conference Board, 1963), p. 21.

A periodical is published at stated intervals—daily, weekly, monthly, quarterly—the issues being numbered in succession. For the most part, each issue is composed of articles by different authors. References to such articles follow the pattern outlined in section 22b, pp. 29-30. For such references, the proper style is not likely to be in question. Occasionally, however, an entire issue of a publication is devoted to one long paper by one author. Sometimes that issue takes the place of the more usual multi-article issue; sometimes it bears a supplementary number. In either case its documentation raises a question: Should it conform to the style of a whole publication or to that of a component part? The answer is in the view taken both by the periodical and by libraries that such a paper is published *in the periodical*. Reference to it, then, should be in the usual style of an article, except that its special designation as shown on the cover of the issue is included in the reference (e.g., supplement, special number).

Elias Folker, "Report on Research in the Capital Markets," Journal of Finance, XXIX, supplement (May, 1964), 15.

(6) *Facts of publication.* As listed under section 22, *a*),
(5) (p. 29), the facts of publication include place
(city), publisher, and date, and, when necessary, total
number of volumes and/or edition.

They should be given for printed books, monographs, and pamphlets, and for materials published in
mimeographed, multigraphed, or other copy-machine
form. But note the following exceptions:

Classical and biblical works	omit	all facts of publication
Legal works and some public documents	usually omit	all but the date
Dictionaries, general encyclopedias, and atlases	omit	all but edition and date
In certain disciplines and in certain fields the citations	omit	name of publisher
Periodicals, in general	omit	all but the date

(*a*) *Number of volumes.* This is required in any reference to a multivolume work as a whole; it may
be included, however, in any reference to the
work. Write, for example, "2 vols.," not "vols. 2"
or "II vols.," and add a semicolon.

(*b*) *Number of edition.* This is necessary for any edition other than the first. Write, for example, "1st
ed., rev." or "1st rev. ed." (observe that they are
not the same), or "2d ed.," and follow with a
semicolon.

Exception: If both the foregoing facts are
given, they may be separated with a comma, and
a semicolon placed after the edition.

(*c*) *Place of publication.* When the names of several

cities appear under the publisher's imprint, give the first, which is the location of the editorial offices, and follow with a colon. If the city is not generally well known, mention the state as well, using the standard abbreviation; for example, "Glencoe, Ill." Identify Cambridge by writing "Cambridge, England" (*never* abbreviate, "Eng."), unless it is followed by "Cambridge University Press"; and "Cambridge, Mass.," unless it is followed by "Harvard University Press." For foreign cities, use the English name if there is one: Cologne, not Köln; Munich, not München; Florence, not Firenze; Padua, not Padova; Milan, not Milano; Rome, not Roma; Prague, not Praha; and so on.

It is permissible, when a title page reads, for example, "Chicago and London," to give both. But do not assume that "and London" should be added in references to works whose title pages do not show it.

When the title page gives no place of publication, write "n.p." (for "no place").

(*d*) *Name of publishing agency.*[1] Follow exactly the style used by the publisher in writing the firm's name, except that "The" at the beginning should be omitted. Note spelling and punctuation and whether such words as "and," "Company," "Brothers" are spelled out or written "&," "Co.," "Bros."

---

[1] The broader term, "publishing agency," rather than "publisher," is used here because some works are published by societies, institutions of learning, commerce, banking, and the like, which are not publishers per se. The terms are used interchangeably in the text of the section.

If the title page indicates that a work was co-published, the citation should indicate both publishers: New York: Alfred A. Knopf and Viking Press, 1966. Boston: Ginn & Co., 1964; Montreal: Round Press, 1964.

The title page of a book issued by a subsidiary of a publishing house gives both names, and any citation of the book should include both: Cambridge: Belknap Press of the Harvard University Press, 1965.

If a work was published for an institution, society, or the like, and their name appears on the title page together with the publisher's name, the references should include both names: New York: Columbia University Press for the American Geographical Society, 1947.

If a work has been reprinted at a later date by a different publisher, the fact will frequently be shown on the entry card for the work in the library card catalog. Such information is especially useful for locating some hard-to-find old works.

Do not substitute the present name of a publishing house for the one appearing on the title page. For example, Harcourt, Brace & World, Inc., should not be used in place of Harcourt, Brace & Co. before 1961.

Do not translate parts of the names of foreign publishers even though the place of publication has been Anglicized (as it should be). Write, for example, "Compagnie" or "Cie.," not "Company" or "Co."; "et Frère," not "and Brother," or "and Bro."

It is acceptable to use the abbreviated forms of

publishers' names as they are listed for American publishers in *Books in Print,* issued annually by R. R. Bowker Co., and for British publishers in the *Reference Catalogue of Current Literature,* published by J. Whitaker & Sons, Ltd.

But follow consistently one style or the other throughout the paper; do not use the full form for some publishers and the abbreviated form for others.

In accordance with long-established practice in certain disciplines and certain fields, their citations omit names of publishers. They appear, for example, "New York, 1965," or "2 vols., 3d ed.; New York, 1965." Note that when the publisher is not given, a comma instead of a colon follows the name of the city.

(*e*) *Date of publication.* The date usually appears on the title page, either with the publisher's imprint, or overleaf in the copyright date. There may be more than one copyright date; if so, the last is the one under which the work was issued. But there may also be one or more dates shown in addition to the copyright date. Since those refer to *reprintings,* or new impressions, not new editions, they should be disregarded. The copyright date is the one to use—unless the date is on the face of the title page.

If no date is shown, write "n.d." (for "no date"): New York: Grosset & Dunlap, n.d. If, however, the date has been established by another means than that of the title page, place the date in brackets: New York: Grosset & Dunlap [1931].

When the reference is to a multivolume work *in its entirety* and it was published over a period of more than one year, the inclusive dates of publication are shown: 1960-65. But if the reference is to only one volume of the work, the date of publication of that volume only is normally given (see sec. 7, below).

For reference to a multivolume work still in progress, the date is followed by a dash: 1960—.

All the facts of publication, in their order as listed in section *a*(5) (p. 29), are placed together between parentheses. Note that when the specific reference (page or volume and page) is cited, it follows the facts of publication and is preceded by a comma. Note, too, that when the facts consist of two items, they are separated with a comma. And, further, that "n.p." may stand for "no place" or for "no publisher," or for both.

References to periodicals omit place and publisher, except that for a foreign periodical of limited circulation the place of publication may well be given.

Jack Fishman, "Un grand homme dans son intimité: Churchill," Historia (Paris), No. 220 (Nov. 1964), pp. 684-94.

(7) *Volume number.* Reference to a work of more than one volume must mention the volume as well as the page number. If the volumes were published in different years, the reference must indicate this fact either by giving inclusive dates of publication and placing the volume number after the facts of publication, as:

Paul Tillich, Systematic Theology (3 vols.; Chicago: University of Chicago Press, 1951-63), I, 45.

or by giving only the publication date of the particular

volume referred to and placing the volume number before the facts of publication.

> Paul Tillich, _Systematic Theology_, I (Chicago: University of Chicago Press, 1951), 45.

Placement of the volume number before the facts of publication is contrary to the style normally used in citing books, but it is permissible in such a case as the one mentioned and it has the advantage of giving the date of the particular volume.

Volume numbers should be expressed in capital Roman numerals, regardless of whether they are expressed in Roman or in Arabic by the works themselves.

References to periodicals other than newspapers and popular magazines (weekly, semi-monthly, or monthly) normally cite the volume number, followed by the month and year, enclosed in parentheses.

> Don Swanson, "Dialogue with a Catalog," _Library Quarterly_, XXXIV (December, 1963), 113-25.

If the volume is followed by the number, only the year need be given: XXXIV, No. 4 (1963).

For those periodicals that have been published in more than one series of volumes, the appropriate series as well as the volume number should be designated, as, for example, Old Series (O.S.), or New Series (N.S.), or 2d Series (2d Ser.).

For newspapers and for popular magazines published weekly or semi-monthly or monthly, volume numbers are normally omitted; those periodicals are most readily identified by their dates.

> Robert Claiborne, "Digging Up Prehistoric America," _Harper's_, April, 1966, pp. 69-74.

(8) *Page number(s)*. Refer to a single page as, for example, "p. 60," and refer to more than one page as, for example, "pp. 60-61," not "pp. 60-1." Similarly, write "pp. 140-42," not "pp. 140-2." If the first digit in the second number is higher than that in the first number, write both numbers in full: "pp. 295-315," not "pp. 295-15."

Use exact page numbers in preference to such a designation as "pp. 80-82ff." (pages 80-82 and following pages). Since "f." refers only to the single page immediately following the number mentioned, it should be avoided. For example, write "pp. 80-81" rather than "pp. 80f."

Passim ("here and there") should be used only in referring to inclusive pages covering a considerable stretch of text or to a chapter or other long part: "pp. 80-95, *passim*." "*Passim*, chap. ii." *Passim* may either follow or precede the specific reference.

(9) *Omission of abbreviations "Vol." and "p."* In a reference including *both* a volume and a page number, the abbreviations "Vol." and "p." or "pp." are usually omitted.

W. T. Jones, <u>A History of Western Philosophy</u> (New York: Harcourt, Brace & Co., 1952), II, 940.

In certain kinds of references, omission of "Vol." and "p." might result in ambiguity. In the following, for example, the volume number is that of the series rather than that of the specific work:

Leonard L. Watkins, <u>Commercial Banking Reform in the United States</u>, Michigan Business Studies, Vol. VIII, No. 5 (Ann Arbor: University of Michigan, 1938), p. 464.

And in the following, the relationship of the two titles

is clearer when the volume number is designated as such.

Gabriel Marcel, <u>The Mystery of Being</u>, Vol. II: <u>Faith and Reality</u> (Chicago: Henry Regnery Co., 1960), p. 19.

When in addition to volume and page some other division of the work is mentioned, that division must be appropriately designated even though the abbreviations "Vol." and "p." are omitted.

Paul Tillich, <u>Systematic Theology</u> (Chicago: University of Chicago Press, 1951-63), I, Part II, 165.

23. *Parts that should be expressed in Roman numerals.*—Capital Roman numerals are used to express volume numbers, except in legal references and in some scientific fields (see chap. ix). They are also used in referring to books, parts (in some cases), divisions, acts (of a play), except as they apply to classical and other ancient works (see sec. 37, p. 50). Lower-case Roman numerals (i, ii, v, ix, etc.) are used in referring to chapters, introductory pages of a book, scenes in a play, and verses of a poem.

24. *Parts that should be expressed in Arabic numerals.*—Arabic numerals are used in referring to pages (other than introductory pages, as indicated above), columns, lines; parts, in some cases; all divisions of classical works; and document numbers in collections of inscriptions, papyri, and ostraca.

25. *Titles that should be underlined and those that should be quoted.*—For the most part, titles of written works, published or unpublished, are either underlined or quoted, depending upon their form. The general rule is to underline the titles of *whole published works*—which in printed matter are italicized—and to quote the titles of *component parts* of whole published works, and the titles of *unpublished works*.

It is important to note that although a published work is usually thought of as being printed, it may be produced by a photo-offset process, such as lithoprinting or planographing, or by one of the multicopy processes, such as mimeographing, multigraphing, or multilithing. If it bears a publisher's imprint, it should be treated as published rather than unpublished material.

a) *Underline* the titles of all the following kinds of published materials: books, pamphlets, bulletins, periodicals (newspapers, magazines, journals); collections of inscriptions, papyri, and ostraca; plays, motion pictures, symphonies, operas; and stories, essays, poems, lectures, sermons, proceedings, and reports when *published separately*. Note that the general title of a multivolume work and also the titles, if any, of the individual volumes are underlined (see examples under i) and j), p. 75).

b) *Quote* the titles of component parts of whole publications: chapters and other divisions of books; articles in periodicals; stories, essays, poems, lectures, sermons, and the like in anthologies or similar collections; short poems and musical compositions; radio and television programs; the English translation of a work in a foreign tongue; and unpublished works such as typed or "processed" reports, lectures, minutes, theses, and dissertations.

26. *Titles that should be neither underlined nor "quoted."*—The names of the books of the Bible and of all sacred scriptures (Koran, Upanishads, Vedanta, etc.) are neither underlined nor quoted.

27. *Capitalization of titles.*—Two methods of capitalization of titles of English works are recognized; but one scheme or the other should be adopted and used consistently throughout the paper, both in the footnote and the bibliographic entries and wherever else the titles appear. The two schemes are:

a) Capitalization of the first and last words, nouns, pronouns, adjectives, adverbs, and verbs.

b) Capitalization of the first word, proper nouns, and proper adjectives.

In the titles of French, Italian, and Spanish works, the first word, all proper nouns, but not the adjectives derived from proper nouns, are capitalized.

In the titles of German works, the first word and all nouns and words used as nouns are capitalized. Of the adjectives derived from nouns, only those derived from the names of persons are capitalized.

An exception to the schemes of capitalization here mentioned may be made in a paper concerned, for example, with a specific edition of a work, or with a manuscript, when the exact manner in which the title appeared is significant.

28. *Split references.*—If at the first mention of a work the author's full name is brought into the text close to the footnote number, it may be omitted in the note. After the first reference, occurrence in the text of the surname alone permits its omission in the note.

Similarly, if both name and title of the work are given in the text, they may be omitted in the note, which then might consist either of the facts of publication and volume and/or page, or of the reference alone.

29. *Abbreviations.*—In footnote and bibliographic materials, a word designating a part of a work may be abbreviated if it is followed by a number. In the list of standard abbreviations below, note that those underlined should always be underlined;

that the kind of numeral (Roman—capital or small—or Arabic) following a part should be the kind used in designating that part; that an abbreviation here capitalized should always be capitalized, but that the others should be capitalized only when they begin a footnote.

```
art. iv (plural, arts.), article
b., born
Bk. I (plural, Bks. In classical references an arabic numeral is
     used), book
c. 220 (plural, cc. [used in law citations only]), chapter
ca. (circa), about
cf., compare
ch. 3 (plural, chs. [used especially in legal citations]),
     chapter
chap. ii (plural, chaps.), chapter
col. 6 (plural, cols.), column
d., died
e.g. (exempli gratia), for example
ed. (plural, edd.), edition
ed. (plural, eds.), editor ("ed." may also be used for
     "edited")
et al. (et alii), and others
et seq. (et sequens; plural, et sqq.), and the following
Fig. 2 (plural, Figs.), figure
fl. (floruit), flourished, i.e., reached greatest development
     or influence
i.e. (id est), that is
ibid. (ibidem), in the same place
idem (never to be abbreviated id.). the same person
infra, below
l. 10 (plural, ll.), line
MS (plural, MSS), manuscript
n. 5 (plural, nn.), note, footnote
n.d., no date
n.n., no name
n.p., no place (may stand also for "no publisher")
No. 12 (plural, Nos.), number
p. (plural, pp.), page
par. (plural, pars.), paragraph
passim, here and there (frequently preceded by et, "and")
Pl. III (plural, Pls.), plate
Pt. II (plural, Pts.), part
q.v. (quod vide), which see
s.v. (sub verbo), under the word
s.v. (sub voce), under the title
sec. 9 (plural, secs.), section
sic, thus
supra, above
trans., translated, translator
```

```
vs. 4 (plural, vss.), verse (in a reference to both verse and
    line, a small Roman numeral refers to the verse)
Vol. II (plural, Vols. when followed by a number; vols. when
    preceded by a number), volume
```

Titles of well-known journals, publications of learned societies, and dictionaries may be abbreviated in capital letters, without spaces or periods, for use in footnotes but not in bibliographic entries.

```
MLN, Modern Language Notes
PMLA, Publications of the Modern Language Association
HDB, Hastings' Dictionary of the Bible
OED, Oxford English Dictionary
```

Also, it is permissible for the writer who must refer frequently to the same work to devise an abbreviation to be used after the first, full reference.

30. *Citation taken from a secondary source.*—For a citation of the work of one author as found in that of another, both the work in which the reference was found (secondary source) and the title of the work mentioned therein must be noted. In general, the style illustrated in footnote 1 should be followed, but if it were more significant for the purposes of the paper to emphasize Hulbert's citing of the *Jesuit Relations*, the style of the second footnote should be used.

```
1Jesuit Relations and Allied Documents, Vol. LIX, n. 41,
quoted in [or "cited by"] Archer Butler Hulbert, Portage Paths
(Cleveland: Arthur H. Clark, 1903), p. 181.
```

Or the reverse form:

```
2Archer Butler Hulbert, Portage Paths (Cleveland: Arthur
H. Clark, 1903), p. 181, quoting [or "citing"] Jesuit Relations
and Allied Documents, Vol. LIX, n. 41.
```

SPECIAL FORMS

31. *Newspapers.*—Although references to newspaper articles may include no more than the name of the paper, the date, and the page number, it is convenient to have the title of the article as well as the name of the writer, if the latter is given. Sunday editions of large metropolitan papers are sometimes printed in separately numbered sections, and in such case the section number must be mentioned. If the name of the newspaper does not include its place of publication, the name should be given in parentheses, except in the cases of such widely circulated newspapers as the *Wall Street Journal* and the *Christian Science Monitor.*

> Robert A. Amen, "Four Million Reside in Mobile Homes," New York Times, Oct. 21, 1962, sec. 8, p. 1R. [Reference to article in a Sunday edition, made up of several sections, separately paged.]

> "Ike Favors More Force in War," Palo Alto Times, Oct. 31, 1966, p. 4. [Reference to article in a daily paper, paged consecutively throughout.]

> Editorial, Wall Street Journal, Nov. 1, 1966, p. 8.

> The Times (London), May 1, 1965, p. 8.

An initial "The" in the title is omitted even though it may appear in the masthead. *The Times* (London) and *The New Yorker* are exceptions.

32. *Encyclopedia articles.*—Reference to a signed article in an encyclopedia is in much the same form as that of an article in a journal. All general encyclopedias have been published in several editions, and the particular edition carrying the article cited must be included in the reference. No new *numbered* editions of either the *Americana* or the *Britannica* have appeared for more than thirty years, but owing to a policy of continuous revision they are reissued annually. Thus it is the *year date* of the edition rather than its number that should be used in most references to articles in those encyclopedias. All editions of the *Britannica* earlier than the fourteenth, however, should be mentioned by number.

J. W. Comyns-Carr, "Blake, William," <u>Encyclopaedia
Britannica</u>, 11th ed., IV, 36-38. [Number of edition, which is
earlier than the 14th, given rather than year date of issue.]

"Falmouth," <u>Encyclopaedia Britannica</u>, 1964, IX, 53.

"Sitting Bull," <u>Encyclopedia Americana</u>, 1962, XXV, 48.

33. *Radio and television programs.*—References vary, depending upon the amount of detail that is included. If the reference is to a program in a series, the series title should be given first. The particular program, participants, etc., may or may not be mentioned. The name of the network is more important than that of the local station.

"Twentieth Century," C.B.S. telecast, Oct. 28, 1962:
"I Remember: Dag Hammarskjöld." Narrator, Walter Cronkite.

34. *Novels.*—Novels, many of which may appear in various editions with different pagination, are best referred to by chapter (or by part or book, and chapter) rather than by page.

Joseph Conrad, <u>Heart of Darkness</u> (New York: Doubleday,
Page & Company, 1903), chap. iii.

35. *Plays and long poems.*—The citing of English classics may be in the same style as that prescribed for Greek and Latin classical works (see sec. 37 below), except that for plays capital Roman numerals indicate acts, small Roman numerals indicate scenes, and Arabic numerals, lines. Facts of publication are omitted.

Shakespeare <u>Romeo and Juliet</u> III.ii.83.

Milton <u>Paradise Lost</u> i.143-45.

References to modern plays are made in the following form:

Louis O. Coxe and Robert Chapman, <u>Billy Budd</u> (Princeton:
Princeton University Press, 1951), I.ii.83.

36. *Shorter poems.*—References to shorter poems, which ordinarily are published in collections, quote the title of the poem, and refer to verses with small Roman numerals and to lines with Arabic numerals, or to either verse or lines if the poem is short.

> Francis Thompson, "The Hound of Heaven," The Oxford Book of Modern Verse (New York: Oxford University Press, 1937), iii.7-10.

37. *Classical works.*—No punctuation is used following the author's name or the title of the work. Abbreviations are widely used for: name of author; title of work; collections of inscriptions, papyri, ostraca, and so on; titles of well-known periodical and reference tools. For a list of accepted abbreviations, the *Oxford Classical Dictionary* should be consulted. It is not recommended, however, that such abbreviations be used except in papers on predominantly classical topics. In Latin and Greek titles, only the first word, proper nouns, and adjectives derived from proper nouns are capitalized. The different levels of division of a work (book, section, line, etc.) are indicated with Arabic numerals, separated with periods except when a succession of parts, sections, or lines is shown. Since classical works in general are found in many editions, facts of publication are usually omitted; but if page numbers are referred to, the edition *must be* mentioned. (See n. 4 below.)

> [1]Cicero De officiis 1. 133, 140.
>
> [2]Homer Odyssey 9. 266-71.
>
> [3]Juvenal Sat. 1. 73.
>
> [4]Horace Satires, Epistles and Ars poetica, Loeb Classical Library (London, 1932), p. 12.

References to collections of inscriptions, papyri, and ostraca use capital Roman numerals for volume numbers. Following the volume number comes the document number in Arabic numerals, with the divisions within the document also expressed in Arabic numerals. Note that commas separate title from volume number, and volume number from document number, after which the different divisions are separated with periods.

IG <u>Rom</u>., III, 739. 9. 10. 17.

<u>POxy</u>., 1485. [No volume number here.]

A superior figure placed either immediately after the title of a work, or after the volume number of a collection and before the following punctuation, indicates the number of the edition.

Stolz-Schmalz <u>Lat. Gram.</u>^{5}, pp. 390-91.

<u>IG</u>, I^2, 1021.

A superior letter or number placed immediately after a number referring to a division of a work indicates a subdivision. If preferred, such letters may be placed on the line, and either capital or small letters may be used in accordance with the source being cited.

Aristotle <u>Metaphysics</u> 3. 3. 996^{b}5-8.
OR:
Aristotle <u>Metaphyics</u> 3. 3. 996b5-8.

38. *Scriptural references.*—The names of the books of the Bible, of the Apocrypha, of the Apocalyptic, and of the versions of the Bible should be abbreviated when exact references are given. Chapter and verse, separated with a colon, are both indicated with Arabic numerals. The word "Bible" is not underlined and neither are the names of the books. The King James version is assumed unless another is indicated.

Psalm 103:6-14.

I Cor. 13:1-3. (R.S.V.)

Non-Christian sacred scriptures are referred to in the same manner as Christian.

39. *Legal citations.*—Law publications use a style of citation very different from that in other fields. Space permits no more than a brief treatment of legal citations here, and the materials chosen for illustration are, therefore, those which it is thought may be most useful to the student. The Harvard Law Review Association publishes a much more complete guide—*A Uniform System of Citation* (10th ed., 1958). The style of reference here set forth follows that guide in most respects; where it differs, the changes are due largely to the fact that this manual is addressed principally to students using a typewriter rather than to those preparing copy for printing.

A conspicuous feature of legal reference usage is that of abbreviations—for names of periodicals and law reports, courts, organs of government, besides those commonly used in footnotes generally. (*A Uniform System* . . . contains a number of lists of such abbreviations.)

The styles of reference given in the examples are those appropriate for footnotes. In the text, and in textual matter in footnotes, names of cases and titles of all publications of whatever kind—books, periodicals, reports, documents, hearings—are underlined. Materials such as periodical titles, which are abbreviated in footnotes, are spelled out in all textual matter.

Papers on topics that are predominantly legal should employ the style of reference discussed in this section, but when papers in other fields refer to books and periodicals in the field of law, as is frequently done in the social sciences, for example, the style of reference to legal works should adapt to that of the topical field in order to preserve a uniform style.

A paper in the field of law may have occasion to refer to government documents other than those mentioned above. In such case, the discussion and examples in chapter viii may be useful. The forms of citation would require change to those common to legal citations.

a) *Court cases*.—Citations of court cases give the name of the case, volume number, name of law report(s), page number, and year date, in that order. For decisions that appear in both an official and an unofficial report, it is proper to cite both, the official report being mentioned first (n. 1). Some early reports are named for court reporters (the names of a few are abbreviated). For a reporter of the United States Supreme Court, "U.S." should appear after the name (n. 2); for a state reporter, the state abbreviation. If "ex parte," "ex rel.," or "in re" forms a part of the case name, that expression is underlined; otherwise there is no underlining in the citation (n. 3).

The court that decided the case must be indicated in the citation. In many instances the name of the report identifies the court, and it is assumed to be the highest in the jurisdiction (n. 4). But most unofficial reports, and all those named for a reporter, do not of themselves indicate the jurisdiction, and both the jurisdiction and the name of the court must be added (n. 5). However, for a case cited to a named reporter, if the court that rendered the decision is the highest of the jurisdiction, only the jurisdiction is mentioned (n. 6). Reference to a case decided by a U.S. court of appeals must indicate the circuit number (n.7).

[1]King v. Order of United Commercial Travelers, 333 U.S. 153, 68 Sup. Ct. 488, 92 L. Ed. 608 (1948).

[2]Collector v. Day, 11 Wall. (U.S.), 113 (1870).

[3]Ex parte Mahone, 30 Ala. 49 (1847).

[4]How v. State, 9 Mo. 690 (1846).

[5]Leary v. Friedenthal, 299 S.W.2d 563 (Mo. Ct. App. 1957).

[6]Morse v. Kieran, 3 Rawle 325 (Pa. 1832).

[7]United States v. Eldridge, 302 F.2d 463 (4th Cir. 1962).

For English court cases the pattern of citation follows in general that of court cases in the United States (n. 8). Although normally the date is given at the end of the citation, for law reports beginning in 1891 and for the *All England Reports*, the date is placed in brackets preceding the series volume and page notation (n. 9). Both the bracketed date (of publication) and the volume number are necessary inasmuch as each series is renumbered yearly (nn. 9, 10). In the case of a *decision date* differing in year from the publication date, the decision date is added at the end of the citation (n. 10).

[8]Comber v. Jones, 3 Bos. & Pull. 114, 127 Eng. Rep. 62 (C.P. 1802).

[9]Fyfe v. Garden, [1946] 1 All E.R. 366 (H.L.).

[10]Lemon v. Lardeur, [1947] 2 All E.R. 329 (C.A. 1946).

b) *Statutory materials.*—Constitutions are cited to article and section (and clause, if relevant) (n. 11). An amendment to the United States Constitution should be mentioned by number, followed by notation of the section (n. 12). Articles of the Constitution are indicated by capital Roman numerals; articles of state constitutions are indicated by capital Roman numerals or Arabic numerals, as the constitutions themselves may show them. Amendments to the federal Constitution are numbered in capital Roman. Sections and clauses are numbered in Arabic. If in a reference

to a portion of a state constitution, that portion has been
significantly amended since the time for which it is cited,
or if it is no longer in force, the date of adoption of the
portion cited is given (n. 14).

[11]U.S. Const. art. I, sec. 5.

[12]U.S. Const. amend. XIV, sec. 2.

[13]Ill. Const. art. 5, sec. 2.

[14]N.Y. Const. art 2, sec. 6 (1894).

Before enactment, Congressional bills and resolutions
are cited:

[15]H.R. 11818, 89th Cong., 1st Sess., sec. 301(a) (1965).

[16]S. Res. 218, 83d Cong., 2d Sess. (1954).

After passage, bills and joint and concurrent resolutions
are cited as statutes. They reach the *U.S. Code* in steps, as
time for publication permits, appearing in the *Congressional
Record* (n. 17) before publication in the *Statutes at Large*
(n. 18), and often in the *U.S. Code Annotated* before the
Code. After publication in the *Code,* statutes should be cited
to the *Code* alone or, as a matter of convenience for the
reader, both to the *Statutes* and the *Code* (n. 19). Many
statutes are cited by popular name as well as official name
(n. 19). Untitled acts are cited as in note 20.

[17]S. Con. Res. 21, 83d Cong., 2d Sess., 100 Cong. Rec.
2929 (1954).

[18]Clayton Act, 64 Stat. 1125 (1950).

[19]Labor Management Relations Act (Taft-Hartley Act),
sec. 301(a), 61 Stat. 156 (1947), 29 U.S.C. sec. 185(a) (1952).
[References to the U.S. Code are always to sections and not
pages.]

[20]Act of July 23, 1947, ch. 302, 61 Stat. 413.

Citations of state laws follow the pattern of federal laws.

[21]Corporate Securities Law, Cal. Corp. Code, secs.
25000-26104.

English statutes are cited by name and chapter, with the
regnal year of the sovereign indicated before his name.

[22]Companies Act, 1948, 19 & 20 George 5, ch. 38.

c) *Government reports, debates, hearings.*—These are cited as
illustrated below. Citations of *hearings* must always indicate the committee, identified as House or Senate (n. 26).

[23]H.R. Rep. No. 871, 78th Cong., 1st Sess. 49 (1943).

[24]Federal Trade Comm'n, Report on Utility Corporations,
S. Doc. No. 92, 70th Cong., 1st Sess., pt. 71A (1935).

[25]100 Cong. Rec. 8820 (1954) (remarks of Senator Blank).
[A citation to the bound edition. The daily edition, which is
differently paged, must be indicated by date, e.g., Feb. 10,
1954.]

[26]Hearings before the House Banking Committee on the
Housing Act of 1949, 81st Cong., 1st Sess., ser. 9, pt. 4 at 109
(1949).

d) *Books and periodicals.*—Authors are cited by surname
alone, unless works are mentioned by more than one author
with the same surname. Volume numbers, expressed in
Arabic numerals, precede the author's name in a book citation (n. 27); they precede the title of a periodical (n. 31).
Page numbers not preceded by "p." ("pp."), follow book
and periodical titles, without punctuation between them.
Facts of publication consist of year date alone, except that
the edition of a book is noted if it is other than the first (n.
27). For a work that is part of a series (numbered or un-
numbered), issued by another than the author, the name of
the series and the number, if any, are noted in parentheses
before the publication date (n. 28). If the title of a work
incorporates the name of the author—whether of a person,
or an official, or an institution—the reference should be

rearranged to cite the author first. If the author is a government official, this fact should be indicated by placing "U.S.," "N.Y.," or "Boston," as appropriate, before the name (n. 30). The title of an article in a periodical or of an essay in the collected works of an author is enclosed in quotation marks (nn. 31, 32). In the latter case, notation of the volume number precedes the author's name (n. 32).

27 2 Holdsworth, A History of English Law 278 (6th ed. 1938).

28 Young, The Contracting Out of Work 145 (Research Ser. No. 1, Queen's University Industrial Centre, 1964).

29 Black, Law Dictionary 85 (4th ed. 1951). [The work is entitled Black's Law Dictionary.]

30 U.S., Comptroller of the Currency, Annual Report, 1935 (1936). [The title of the work is Annual Report of the Comptroller of the Currency, 1935.]

31 Hutcheson, "A Case for Three Judges," 48 Harv. L. Rev. 795 (1934).

32 4 Bentham, "Panopticon," Works 122-24 (1893).

e) *Loose-leaf services.*—These services, which compile such information as statistical texts, regulations and rulings, editorial comment, recent cases, and citations to other pertinent authorities, frequently require citation. Reference is to the name of the service, omitting the publisher's name unless the omission would cause confusion. If the service is revised annually, the year date must be included. Paragraphs rather than pages are given.

33 2 P-H 1966 Fed. Tax Serv. para. 10182.

40. *Manuscript collections.*—The location, title, and number (or similar designation) should be given. If a specific document or letter is referred to, it should be mentioned either at the beginning or the end of the note, as in notes 2 and 3 below.

[1] British Museum, Arundel MSS, 285, fol. 165b.

[2] Great Britain, Public Record Office MSS, Foreign Office, Egypt, Vol. II, Petition of Briggs, Feb. 8, 1806.

[3] Letter, A. H. Strong to W. R. Harper, Dec. 23, 1890, University of Chicago, Archives, Harper Letter File.

41. *Miscellaneous unpublished materials.*—Because of their variety, such materials are cited in different forms. If the material has a title, that title is placed within quotation marks, following the name of the sponsoring organization or of the author, if any. If there is a descriptive title, it is not quoted. Mention of the nature of the material follows the title, and although exact location can seldom be given, the citation should include information which would permit the material to be found. The information given about a personal letter may be much or little, depending upon its value as source material (see nn. 1 and 2).

[1] John Blank, personal letter.

[2] Letter from Alan Cranston, California State Controller, Sacramento, Oct. 22, 1962.

[3] Morristown (Kanasas) Orphans' Home, Minutes of Meetings of the Board of Managers, Meeting of May 6, 1930.

[4] Sidney E. Mead, "Some Eternal Greatness," sermon preached at the Rockefeller Chapel, University of Chicago, July 31, 1960.

[5] O. C. Phillips, Jr., "The Influence of Ovid on Lucan's Bellum civile" (unpublished Ph.D. dissertation, University of Chicago, 1962), p. 14.

42. *Interviews.*—The person or group interviewed, place, and date are noted.

A. A. Wyller, private interview held during meeting of the American Astronomical Society, Pasadena, Calif., June, 1964.

Farmers' State Bank, Barrett, Neb., interviews with a selected list of depositors, August, 1960.

SECOND OR LATER REFERENCES

When a work has once been cited in complete form, later references to it should be in shortened form.

43. *References using "ibid."*—When references to the same work follow each other without any intervening reference, even though separated by several pages, the abbreviation *ibid.* (for the Latin *ibidem,* "in the same place") is used to repeat as much of the preceding reference as is appropriate for the new entry.

[1]Wilbur L. Cross, The History of Henry Fielding (2d ed.; New Haven: Yale University Press, 1918), I, 49. [A first, and therefore complete, reference to the work.]

[2]Ibid. [With no intervening reference, a second reference to the same volume and page of Cross's work requires only ibid.]

[3]Ibid., II, 51. [Here another volume and page number of Cross's work is referred to.]

Ibid. may also be used to repeat the title of a journal in the immediately preceding reference if the author is the same; the title of the article may be different.

[4]Sune V. Main, "Matthew 10: An Interpretation," Journal of the New Testament, XXXVII (June, 1918), 37.

[5]Sune V. Main, "The First Epistle to the Corinthians," ibid., XXXIX (June, 1920), 84.

But *ibid.* should not be used to refer to the last-named work in the immediately preceding footnote if that footnote cited two or more works.

If a number of pages separate the references to a given work, the writer may prefer, for the sake of clarity, to repeat the title rather than to use *ibid.* even though no reference to another work has intervened.

Since *ibid.* means "in the same *place,*" it must not be employed to repeat the author's name alone when this is the only item remaining unchanged from the footnote immediately preceding. In such cases the repetition of the author's name is preferred style, although *idem* (meaning "the same person") may be used. *Idem* should not be abbreviated to *id*.

> [1]Arthur Waley, <u>The Analects of Confucius</u> (London: George Allen & Unwin, 1938), p. 33.

Wrong:
> [2]<u>Ibid., Chinese Poems</u> (London: George Allen & Unwin, 1946), p. 51.

> [1]Arthur Waley, <u>The Analects of Confucius</u> (London: George Allen & Unwin, 1938), p. 33.

Right:
> [2]Arthur Waley, <u>Chinese Poems</u> (London: George Allen & Unwin, 1946), p. 51.

44. *References using title.*—Reference to a work which already has been cited in full form, *but not in the reference immediately preceding*, should give the author's last name (but not the first name or initials unless works by two or more persons with the same last name have been cited previously); the title of the work, whether it is that of a whole publication or of a component part; and the specific reference (page, or volume and page, if necessary). The title may be shortened (see subsecs. *a*) and *b*) below).

In footnote references to works previously cited in full, scholarly practice of long standing has used the Latin abbreviations *ibid., op. cit.*, and *loc. cit.* as space savers. An alternate scheme has been to drop *op. cit.* or *loc. cit.* and use only the author's surname with the relevant notation of page(s).

But either scheme may be a stumbling block to the zealous reader. He may have been introduced to a great many authors and titles of their works before meeting "Gates, *op. cit.*, p. 40" in footnote 80. With no notion of what work *op. cit.* represents, he turns first to the bibliography, only to find two or more works

listed for Gates. Nothing for it, then, but to examine all the preceding citations. If he is lucky, he may not go far before locating the original citation. But he may not be lucky; he may have to go back to the beginning; he may even discover that the writer has mentioned two works by Gates, or none at all! One of the pitfalls of rearranging text—and rearranging is probably more common than uncommon—is keeping the footnotes in order, especially making certain that abbreviated forms do not appear before their corresponding full forms. Should the writer slip up, if he has used the style of abbreviated reference that includes the title rather than *op. cit.* or *loc. cit.*, the work will be identifiable—at least to the extent that any additional information desired by the reader can be found in the bibliography. The writer, the reader, the typist—all stand to gain in the use of this unambiguous form.

[1]Philip H. Ashby, <u>History and Future of Religious Thought: Christianity, Hinduism, Buddhism, Islam</u> (Englewood Cliffs, N.J.: Prentice-Hall, Inc., 1963), p. 43.

[2]T. R. V. Murti, <u>The Central Philosophy of Buddhism</u> (London: George Allen & Unwin, Ltd., 1955), pp. 127-28.

[3]<u>Ibid</u>., p. 130. [Reference to a different page of the citation immediately preceding.]

[4]Mircea Eliade, "History of Religions and a New Humanism," <u>History of Religions</u>, I, No. 1 (Summer, 1961), 5.

[5]Ashby, <u>Religious Thought</u>, p. 75. [Another reference to the work cited in n. 1. Other references having intervened, <u>ibid</u>. must not be used. Note the shortened title.]

[6]Murti, <u>Buddhism</u>, p. 140. [Another reference to the work cited in n. 2, using a shortened title.]

[7]Eliade, "History of Religions," pp. 6-7. [Another reference to the journal article cited in n. 4. Note that it uses a shortened form of the title of the article.]

a) Form. Footnotes 5, 6, and 7 above are abbreviated references to works earlier cited in full. It is worth noting that footnote 7, which gives the *title of the article* previously cited and omits the name of the periodical, represents a change from the style specified in earlier editions of this *Manual*. In the abbreviated form that is used whenever *ibid.* is not appropriate, the title in every case should be that of the *specific work*. Note what this means when a particular volume of a multivolume work is mentioned.

Included are:
- surname of author (without first name or initials unless another author with the same surname has been mentioned earlier)
- title of specific work
- page(s)

Omitted are:
- name of author or editor of multivolume work
- over-all title of multivolume work
- name of series
- volume number (unless the *particular work* is in more than one volume)
- number of edition (unless more than one edition has been cited previously)

Consider the following example of a first citation:

Albert C. Baugh, ed., <u>A Literary History of England,</u> Vol. II: <u>The Renaissance (1500-1660),</u> by Tucker Brooke (New York: Appleton-Century-Crofts, Inc., 1948), p. 104.

and a later reference to *Volume II of the multivolume work*:

Brooke, <u>The Renaissance,</u> p. 230. [Since this title is Vol. II of the <u>whole</u> work, volume number should not be mentioned in the reference.]

Now look at the following examples:

Gerald E. Bentley, <u>The Jacobean and Caroline Stage,</u> Vols. I-II: <u>Dramatic Companies and Players</u> (Oxford: Clarendon Press, 1941), I, 24-25.

Bentley, <u>Companies and Players,</u> I, 28. [Here the particular work cited is in two volumes; so volume number is necessary to locate the citation.]

It has been seen that later references to articles in periodicals cite the title of the article, with relevant page numbers, but not the periodical, volume number, or date. Similarly, later references to essays, lectures, stories, poems, or the like, published in anthologies or other collections mention the story (or other component part), but not the anthology.

> Original citation: E. M. Forster, "The Celestial Omnibus," in Fifty Years, Being a Retrospective Collection . . . , selected, assembled, and edited, with an Introduction by Clifton Fadiman (New York: Alfred A. Knopf, 1965), pp. 578-90.

> Later reference: Forster, "Celestial Omnibus," p. 588.

b) *Shortened titles.* In general, titles of from two to five words should not be shortened, but length of the words may be considered and such a title as the following may be shortened as indicated.

Perspectives in American Catholicism   American Catholicism

A shortened title uses the key words of the main title, omitting an initial "A," "An," or "The." Titles beginning with such words as "A Dictionary of," "Readings in," "An Index to," should omit those words for the most part, using the topic as the short title.

A Guide to Rehabilitation of   Handicapped
the Handicapped

Bibliography of North American   Folklore and Folksong
Folklore and Folksong

But occasionally a dictionary or bibliography covers a variety of topics, so that a shortened title would belie its name if all were mentioned. Consider, for example, *An Index to General Literature, Biographical, Historical, and Literary Essays and Sketches, Reports and Publications of Boards and Societies Dealing with Education.*
The only reasonable shortened title is simply *Index.*

Following are examples of full titles with suitable shortened titles.

The Rise of the Evangelical Conception of the Ministry in America	Ministry in America
The American Dream of Destiny and Democracy	American Dream OR Destiny and Democracy
Creation Legends of the Ancient Near East	Creation Legends
Classification and Identification of Handwriting	Handwriting

Do not change the order of the words of the original title or change the form of the words. For example,

Creation Legends of the Ancient Near East	should not be shortened to Near Eastern Legends

When a shortened title is to be used in later reference, the first full citation should indicate the fact: "(Hereinafter referred to as _____.)"

CONTENT FOOTNOTES AND CROSS-REFERENCES

45. *Content footnotes.*—These sometimes consist entirely of the writer's explanation or amplification of the discussion in the text. More often than not, however, the material there presented is supported by references to works or to other parts of the same paper (cross-references). Any one of several ways of placing the references is permissible. The same scheme need not be followed throughout the paper, and in any given note the position which seems most appropriate may be selected. But for references coming at the ends of sentences, either the scheme of enclosing or that of not enclosing in parentheses should be followed consistently. Whether the reference is given in its full form or in abbreviated form will depend upon whether the work has been cited previously. Once the abbreviated title for a given work has been used, it should not be altered.

[1]Professor D. T. Suzuki brings this out with great clarity in his discussions of "stopping" and "no-mindedness"; see, e.g., his chapter on "Swordsmanship" (<u>Zen Buddhism and Its Influence on Japanese Culture</u> [Kyoto: Eastern Buddhist Society, 1938]).

[2]Ernst Cassirer takes important notice of this in <u>Language and Myth</u> (New York: Harper & Bros., 1946), pp. 59-62, and offers a searching analysis of man's regard for things on which his power of inspirited action may crucially depend.

[3]A viewpoint on special librarianship is presented by the author in "The Education of a Catalyst," <u>Special Libraries,</u> LV (October, 1964), 285-89.

46. *Cross-references.*—These are used to refer to other parts of the paper, but never in place of *ibid.* or a reference consisting of author's name and title of the work. *Supra* or *infra* ("above" or "below") may be employed, however, to refer to the *comment* in a content footnote as well as to textual material. The following is an illustration.

> This does not imply that these matters should not be considered when deciding whether it is appropriate to finance a particular government expenditure by debt or by taxes (see <u>supra,</u> pp. 120-22 and n. 2, p. 125).

A cross-reference is often merely to an earlier or a later page— "*Supra*, p. 9" or its English equivalent, "Above, p. 9." Use consistently either the Latin or the English terms.

47. *Quotations in footnotes.*—Quoted matter in footnotes—both that run into the text and that set off from the text of the note— must be enclosed in double quotation marks.

VI

Bibliography

48. *Heading.*—The bibliography[1] lists the sources used in the writing of the paper—not necessarily every work examined but those that were found relevant. The quoting of pertinent passages from works dealing primarily with subjects different from the subject of the paper does not warrant the inclusion of those works in the bibliography.

Since a bibliography rarely includes all that has been written upon a given topic, it is advisable to choose a heading that more accurately represents its contents. Such, for example, are "Selected Bibliography," "Works Cited," and "Sources Consulted." The last is especially suitable if the list includes such sources as personal interviews, lectures, tape recordings, radio or television broadcasts, which for the sake of convenience are by common usage included in a bibliography.

49. *Classification.*—Unless the bibliography is very short, it is usually classified. Among the more common schemes is that of division according to the types of source materials used; another is that of works about an author and works by the same author; another, that of periods of activity. There are many possible bases of classification, and the topic of the paper, its order of presentation, and its thesis sometimes suggest a particular arrangement—possibly one that is unique.

[1] Sample bibliographic entries are shown in chapter vii.

Sometimes the variety of source materials calls for subdivisions of the main classes, with subheadings which may be numbered or lettered.

Within the divisions and subdivisions, the entries should be arranged in a definite order. Although alphabetic order by surname of author is the most common, for some papers another order—for example, chronological—is more helpful. If a scheme other than alphabetic is used, it should be explained in a note.

50. *General form of entries.*—Although the items of information and the order in which they are mentioned are in general the same for bibliographic entries as for footnotes in their full form, there are differences stemming from their contrasting placement, emphasis, and purpose. In the footnote, the author's name is given in the natural order because there is no reason to use reverse order; in the bibliographic entry, the surname is mentioned first because the bibliography is ordinarily arranged in alphabetic order by surnames of authors, and even if it is not so arranged, it is a convenience to show the surname first. Since a primary purpose of the footnote is to give the specific location of the source from which a statement in the text is drawn, volume and page are included; and since it is logical to link page number with name of author and title of the work, the loose separation with commas is employed, and the minor importance of the facts of publication is shown by their insertion within parentheses. On the other hand, the primary purpose of the bibliographic entry is to identify the *whole work* as distinct from a specific part. The importance of all three main items of information—author, title, facts of publication—is shown by separating them with periods and by dropping the parentheses enclosing the facts of publication. Notice, however, that references to periodicals usually retain the parentheses around the month and year, which are normally necessary completely to identify the volume number.

51. *Author's name—some guides in alphabetizing.*—The writing of certain names in reverse order presents problems that are not present when writing them in normal order.

a) Notice how the following names of persons in a succession are written when the surname comes first:

Arthur P. Brownell, Jr.   Brownell, Arthur P., Jr.
Ira Raymond Edwards III   Edwards, Ira Raymond III

b) Names beginning with "M'," "Mc," or "Mac," are listed as though the prefix were spelled "Mac." Similarly, names beginning with "St." or "Ste" are alphabetized as though they began with "Saint" or "Sainte."

c) The first name of the compound governs the placing of compound names. Thus Theodore Watts-Dunton's name is listed under: Watts-Dunton, Theodore.

d) Germanic names spelled with an umlaut are alphabetized as though "ä" were "ae," "ö" were "oe," and "ü" were "ue."

e) English names with prefixes are alphabetized according to the prefix.

à Beckett, Gilbert   O'Flaherty, Liam
De Forest, Lockwood   Van de Graaf, Robert
Du Bois, William   Van Doren, Carl

f) French, Italian, Spanish, and Portuguese names with prefixes consisting either of an article or of a preposition and an article forming one word are alphabetized under the prefix.

Du Moncel   Dall'Ongaro
La Fontaine   Del Rio
Lo Yatto   Della Casa

But if the prefix is a preposition alone, alphabetization is under the name.

Caulaincourt, de   Farina, da

And (in French) if the prefix consists of a preposition and an article that are separated, alphabetization is under the article: La Fontaine, de.

g) Flemish, Swedish, German, and Dutch names are alphabetized under the name, not the prefix:

```
Brink, Bernhard ten        Meer, Jan van der
Bülow, Wilhelm von         Noort, Adam van
Geijerstam, Gustaf af      Stolberg, Christian zu
Hoff, Jacob van't
```

h) There are exceptions to the foregoing, and in case of doubt it is well to consult an encyclopedia or a biographical dictionary.

i) Spanish names which consist of given name (or names) and paternal name and maternal name joined with the conjunction *y* are alphabetized under the paternal name. With this rule in mind alphabetization would be simple, but actually many names omit the conjunction, and in such a name as Manuel Ramón Albeniz, one does not know whether the father's surname is Ramón or whether it is a second given name. The facts must be determined before the name can be entered in the bibliography.

j) Writers who have adopted a religious name sometimes write under that name alone, preceded by the appropriate title. Sometimes they add the surname to the religious name.

```
Hayden, Cuthbert, Father        Eva Catherine, Sister
```

k) Names of authors who have titles of nobility are variously written, depending upon the rank and, for some titles, upon the country as well. Further, for married women the way the name is written depends upon whether the lady holds her title because of her father's rank and/or acquired it through marriage to a nobleman. Note the following:

```
Montagu, Lady Mary (Pierrepont) Wortley [Daughter of a duke;
  married a commoner]
Duff-Gordon, Lucie (Austin) Lady [Title by marriage]
```

Added to titles of nobility in some cases are law or military or ecclesiastical titles.

```
Montgomery of Alamein, Field-Marshal Viscount Bernard Law
```

Some authors are better known under their family names than by their titles and should therefore be listed under the family name, followed by notation of the title.

```
Bacon, Francis, Viscount St. Albans
Walpole, Horace, Earl of Orford
```

For English noblemen other than baronets and knights, the name by which the title is known comes first, followed by the family name. The wife of a peer takes the title corresponding to that of her husband.

```
Wellington, Arthur Wellesley, First Duke of
Russell, Bertrand Arthur William Russell, Third Earl
Browne, Sir Thomas [Knight]
Devonshire, Georgiana (Spencer) Cavendish, Duchess of
```

Limitations of space allow for only a minimum of information on a topic that occupies much shelf space in libraries. In case of doubt, a biographical dictionary should be consulted.

m) In entering authors of the same surname, give first those identified by initials and follow with those whose first given names have the same initial as the name identified by initials alone.

```
Adams, J. B.
Adams, John
Adams, John Quincy
```

n) Successive entries of works by the same author substitute an eight-space line ending with a period for the author's name. If a work is to be listed by the same author in collaboration with another, place such an entry after the works of the author alone, using the following form:

_____, and Blank, Robert John

o) The works of anonymous authors are alphabetized under their titles, not as though their authors were named "Anonymous." Anonymous works for which the names of known or of presumed authors are supplied in brackets are entered under those names.

p) Pseudonymous works are entered under the pseudonyms.

52. *Capitalization and underlining of titles.*—Capitalization must agree with the scheme adopted for the citing of titles in footnotes and elsewhere in the paper (see sec. 27, pp. 44-45).

In the bibliography underlining of the titles of whole publications—books, periodicals, and all other works whose titles are underlined in footnotes—is optional. The quoting of titles of articles and of component parts of whole publications is necessary. Foreign words and phrases must be underlined, except that titles entirely in a foreign language are not underlined if the option is taken of not underlining the titles of whole publications. Nor is a quoted title entirely in a foreign language underlined.

53. *Notation of total number of pages.*—Some institutions and some departments may require that entries of books and pamphlets include the total number of pages in each work. If there is such a notation, it should indicate the preliminary pages and the pages of text separately, e.g., "Pp. xiv+450." For periodical articles, the inclusive pages should be shown.

54. *Indention.*—For ease of reference it is desirable that the author's name should stand out, and prominence is given by placing the name flush with the margin and indenting succeeding lines of each entry a definite number of spaces, observing the same indention for all entries. In general, indention of from four to eight spaces is satisfactory.

If desired, the authors' names can be given further prominence by typing in capitals throughout.

55. *Spacing.*—This may be either double, single, or one and one-half. If single, there should be a double space between entries.

56. *Annotation.*—If the bibliographic entries are annotated, the annotation should be typed in single spacing and should begin on the line following the entry proper. Annotation is not required for all entries.

```
Thompson, Oscar, ed.  International Cyclopedia of Music and Mu-
     sicians.  New York:  Dodd, Mead & Co., 1938.
          An admirable work which brings Grove up to date
     and deals adequately with contemporary music and Ameri-
     can composers.
```

VII

Sample Footnote References and Corresponding Bibliographic Entries

57. The following examples illustrate footnote and bibliographic forms exclusive of those used in citations of public documents and in scientific fields, both of which are discussed hereinafter (see chaps. viii and ix).

The abbreviations "N." and "B." stand, respectively, for footnote entry and bibliographic entry.

BOOKS

a) One author:

N.   ¹Leonard Woolf, <u>Beginning Again</u> (London: Hogarth Press, 1964), p. 185.

B.   Woolf, Leonard.   <u>Beginning Again.</u>   London: Hogarth Press, 1964.

b) Two authors:

N.   ²Walter E. Houghton and G. Robert Stange, <u>Victorian Poetry and Poetics</u> (Cambridge, Mass.: Harvard University Press, 1959), p. 27.

B. Houghton, Walter E., and Stange, G. Robert. _Victorian Poetry and Poetics._ Cambridge, Mass.: Harvard University Press, 1959.

c) *Three authors:*

N. [3]Bernard R. Berelson, Paul F. Lazarsfeld, and William N. McPhee, _Voting_ (Chicago: University of Chicago Press, 1954), pp. 93-103.

B. Berelson, Bernard R.; Lazarsfeld, Paul F.; and McPhee, William N. _Voting._ Chicago: University of Chicago Press, 1954.

d) *More than three authors:*

N. [4]Albert J. Reiss, Jr., _et al._ [Or Albert J. Reiss, Jr., and others], _Occupations and Social Status_ (New York: Free Press of Glencoe, 1961), p. 9.

B. Reiss, Albert J., Jr.; Duncan, Otis Dudley; Hatt, Paul K.; and North, Cecil C. _Occupations and Social Status._ New York: Free Press of Glencoe, 1961.

e) *No author given:*

N. [5]_The Lottery_ (London: J. Watts [1732]), pp. 20-25.

B. _The Lottery._ London: J. Watts [1732].

f) *No author given; name supplied:*

N. [6][Henry K. Blank], _Art for Its Own Sake_ (Chicago: Nonpareil Press, 1910), p. 8.

B. [Blank, Henry K.] _Art for Its Own Sake._ Chicago: Nonpareil Press, 1910.

g) *Pseudonymous author; real name supplied:*

N. [7]Mrs. Markham [Mrs. Elizabeth Cartright Penrose], _A History of France_ (London: John Murray, Ltd., 1872), p. 9.

B. Markham, Mrs. [Mrs. Elizabeth Cartright Penrose.] _A History of France._ London: John Murray, Ltd., 1872.

h) *Association, institution, or the like, as "author":*

N. [8]Special Libraries Association, _Directory of Busi-_

ness and Financial Services (New York: Special Libraries
Association, 1963), p. 21.

B.   Special Libraries Association. Directory of Business and
     Financial Services. New York: Special Libraries
     Association, 1963.

i) *Author's work contained in his collected works:*

N.   9Samuel Taylor Coleridge, Aids to Reflection, in The
Complete Works of Samuel Taylor Coleridge, ed. by W. G. T.
Shedd, I (New York: Harper & Bros., 1884), 209.

B.   Coleridge, Samuel Taylor. Aids to Reflection. The Complete
     Works of Samuel Taylor Coleridge. Edited by W. G. T.
     Shedd. Vol. I. New York: Harper & Bros., 1884.

j) *Separately titled volume in a multivolume work with a general title and editor:*

N.   10J. H. Latané, America as a World-Power, 1897-1907,
Vol. XXV of The American Nation: A History, ed. by A. B.
Hart (28 vols.; New York: Harper & Bros., 1904-18), p. 220.

B.   Latané, J. H. America as a World-Power, 1897-1907. Vol.
     XXV of The American Nation: A History. Edited by
     A. B. Hart. 28 vols. New York: Harper & Bros.,
     1904-18.

k) *Component part by one author in a work edited by another:*

N.   11Paul Tillich, "Being and Love," in Moral Principles of Action, ed. by Ruth N. Anshen (New York: Harper &
Bros., 1952), p. 663.

B.   Tillich, Paul. "Being and Love." Moral Principles of
     Action. Edited by Ruth N. Anshen. New York:
     Harper & Bros., 1952.

m) *Editor in place of author; same form used for compiler:*

N.   12J. N. D. Anderson, ed., The World's Religions
     (London: Inter-Varsity Fellowship, 1950), p. 143.

B.   Anderson, J. N. D., ed. The World's Religions. London:
     Inter-Varsity Fellowship, 1950.

n) Author's work translated by another; same form used if edited:

N.   [13]Ivar Lissner, The Living Past, trans. by J. Maxwell Brownjohn (New York: G. P. Putnam's Sons, 1957), p.
68.

B. Lissner, Ivar. The Living Past. Translated by J. Maxwell
            Brownjohn. New York: G. P. Putnam's Sons, 1957.

o) Multivolume work under general title, with each volume separately titled:

N.   [14]Will Durant, The Story of Civilization, Vol. I:
Our Oriental Heritage (New York: Simon and Schuster, Inc.,
1942), p. 88.

B. Durant, Will. The Story of Civilization. Vol. I: Our Ori-
            ental Heritage. New York: Simon and Schuster,
            Inc., 1942.

p) Part of a series:

N.   [15]Muriel W. Pumphrey, The Teaching of Values and
Ethics in Social Work Education, The Social Work Curriculum
Study, Vol.III (New York: Council on Social Work Education,
1959), p. 25.

B. Pumphrey, Muriel W. The Teaching of Values and Ethics in
            Social Work Education. The Social Work Curriculum
            Study, Vol. III. New York: Council on Social Work
            Education, 1959.

q) Paperback series:

N.   [16]Eric Wolf, Sons of the Shaking Earth, Phoenix
Books (Chicago: University of Chicago Press, 1962), p. 25.

B. Wolf, Eric. Sons of the Shaking Earth. Phoenix Books.
            Chicago: University of Chicago Press, 1962.

r) Book in a foreign language with English title supplied:

N.   [17]Maria Turlejska, Rok Przed Kleska ("The Year Before the Defeat") (Warsaw: Wiedza Powszechna, 1962), p.
445.

B. Turlejska, Maria. Rok Przed Kleska. ("The Year before the
            Defeat.") Warsaw: Wiedza Powszechna, 1962.

s) Book privately printed:

N.   [18]John G. Barrow, A Bibliography of Bibliographies

in Religion (Austin, Texas: By the Author, 716 Brown Bldg.,
1965), p. 25. [City address not always included.]

B.   Barrow, John G. A Bibliography of Bibliographies in Reli-
              gion. Austin, Texas: By the Author, 716 Brown
              Bldg., 1955.

t)   Edition other than the first:

N.   [19]William R. Shepherd, Historical Atlas (8th ed.;
     New York: Barnes and Noble, 1956), p. 10.

B.   Shepherd, William R. Historical Atlas. 8th ed. New York:
              Barnes and Noble, 1956.

REPORTS—PUBLISHED

a)   Author named:

N.   [1]Marcus Pease, Housing for Retired Persons, Report
     to the Mayor's Committee, Sample, Calif., April 20, 1958
     (Sample, Calif: Office of the Mayor, 1958), p. 3.

B.   Pease, Marcus. Housing for Retired Persons. Report to the
              Mayor's Committee, Sample, Calif., April 20, 1958.
              Sample, Calif.: Office of the Mayor, 1958.

b)   Chairman of committee named:

N.   [2]Report of the Commmittee on Financial Institutions
     to the President of the United States, Walter W. Heller,
     chairman (Washington, D.C.: Government Printing Office,
     1963), p. 12.

B.   Report of the Committee on Financial Institutions to the
              President of the United States. Walter W. Heller,
              chairman. Washington, D.C.: Government Printing
              Office, 1963.

c)   Association, board, commission, or the like, the "author":

N.   [3]Commission on Money and Credit, Report of the Com-
     mission, Money and Credit (Englewood Cliffs, N.J.:
     Prentice-Hall, Inc., 1961), p. 167.

B.   Commission on Money and Credit. Report of the Commission.
              Money and Credit. Englewood Cliffs, N.J.:
              Prentice-Hall, Inc., 1961.

PROCEEDINGS

N.   [1]Industrial Relations Research Association. Pro-
     ceedings of Third Annual Meeting (Madison, Wis., 1951),
     p. 30.

B.   Industrial Relations Research Association. <u>Proceedings of Third Annual Meeting</u>. Madison, Wis., 1951.

YEARBOOKS

a) *Department of government:*

N.   [1]U.S., Department of Agriculture, <u>Yearbook of Agriculture, 1941</u> (Washington, D.C.: Government Printing Office, 1941), p. 683.

B.   U.S. Department of Agriculture. <u>Yearbook of Agriculture, 1941</u>. Washington, D.C.: Government Printing Office, 1941.

b) *Article in a yearbook:*

N.   [1]G. M. Wilson, "A Survey of the Social and Business Use of Arithmetic," <u>Second Report of the Committee on Minimal Essentials in Elementary-School Subjects</u>, Sixteenth Yearbook of the National Society for the Study of Education, Part I (Bloomington, Ill.: Public School Publishing Co., 1917), pp. 20-22.

B.   Wilson, G. M. "A Survey of the Social and Business Use of Arithmetic." <u>Second Report of the Committee on Minimal Essentials in Elementary-School Subjects</u>. Sixteenth Yearbook of the National Society for the Study of Education, Part I. Bloomington, Ill.: Public School Publishing Co., 1917.

ARTICLES IN JOURNALS OR MAGAZINES

a) *Article in a journal:*

N.   [1]Barbara K. Varley, "Socialization in Social Work Education," <u>Social Work</u>, VIII (July, 1963), 105.

B.   Varley, Barbara K. "Socialization in Social Work Education." <u>Social Work</u>, VIII (July, 1963), 103-9.

b) *Article in a magazine:*

N.   [2]S. L. A. Marshall, "The Fight at Monkey," <u>Harper's Magazine</u>, November, 1966, pp. 111-22.

B.   Marshall, S. L. A. "The Fight at Monkey." <u>Harper's Magazine</u>, November, 1966, pp. 111-22.

ARTICLE IN AN ENCYCLOPEDIA

a) *Signed article:*

N.   [1]J. W. Comyns-Carr, "Blake, William," Encyclopaedia Britannica, 11th ed., IV, 36-38.

B.   Comyns-Carr, J. W. "Blake, William." Encyclopaedia Britannica. 11th ed. Vol. IV.

b) *Unsigned article:*

N.   [2]"Sitting Bull," Encyclopedia Americana, 1962, XXV, 48.

B.   "Sitting Bull." Encyclopedia Americana. 1962. Vol. XXV.

ARTICLE IN A NEWSPAPER

N.   [1]Editorial, Wall Street Journal, Nov. 1, 1966, p. 8.

B.   Wall Street Journal. Editorial, Nov. 1, 1966.

In the foregoing references to articles in periodicals and encyclopedias, the form of the corresponding bibliographic entry assumes in each case only a single reference to the publication. If the paper has referred to a particular publication more than once, the entry to that publication in the bibliography should indicate it. In some instances the dates of the issues used should be given; in cases where the files of a periodical have been examined for a period of time, the inclusive dates should be set down. For encyclopedias, the issues used should be mentioned. As noted earlier, the entries of general reference works and of periodicals do not include names of editors and publishers.

Wall Street Journal, May 1-10, July 24-28, December 15-18, 1964.

The Times (London), January 4-December 31, 1964.

Saturday Review, July 2, 16, 30, August 6, 20, 27, 1966.

BOOK REVIEWS

N.   [1]Thomas G. Bergin, "In the Days of Knights," review of The Crusades, by Zoé Oldenbourg, in the Saturday Review, July 2, 1966, p. 21.

B.   Bergin, Thomas G. "In the Days of Knights." Review of
      The Crusades, by Zoé Oldenbourg. Saturday Review,
      July 2, 1966, p. 21.

MANUSCRIPT COLLECTIONS

N.   [1]Great Britain, Public Record Office MSS, Foreign
      Office, Egypt, Vol. II, Petition of Briggs, Feb. 8, 1806.

B.   Great Britain. Public Record Office MSS. Foreign Office,
      Egypt, Vol. II.

N.   [2]Letter, A. H. Strong to W. R. Harper, Dec. 23,
      1890, University of Chicago, Archives, Harper Letter File.

B.   University of Chicago. Archives, Harper Letter File.

UNPUBLISHED MATERIALS

N.   [1]O. C. Phillips, Jr., "The Influence of Ovid on
      Lucan's Bellum civile" (unpublished Ph.D. dissertation,
      University of Chicago, 1962), p. 14.

B.   Phillips, O. C., Jr. "The Influence of Ovid on Lucan's
      Bellum civile." Unpublished Ph.D. dissertation,
      University of Chicago, 1962.

N.   [2]American Institute of Planners, Chicago Chapter,
      "Regional Shopping Centers Planning Symposium," Chicago,
      1942, pp. 10-13. (Mimeographed.)

B.   American Institute of Planners, Chicago Chapter. "Regional
      Shopping Centers Planning Symposium," Chicago, 1942.
      (Mimeographed.)

N.   [3]H. P. Luhn, "Keyword-in-Context Index for Technical
      Literature" (paper presented at the 136th meeting of the
      American Chemical Society, Atlantic City, N.J., Sept. 14,
      1959), p. 3.

B.   Luhn, H. P. "Keyword-in-Context Index for Technical Litera-
                    ture." Paper presented at the 136th meeting of the
                    American Chemical Society, Atlantic City, N.J.,
                    Sept. 14, 1959.

N. [4]Morristown (Kansas) Orphans' Home, Minutes of Meetings of the Board of Managers, meeting of May 6, 1950. (Typewritten.)

B. Morristown (Kansas) Orphans' Home. Minutes of Meetings of the Board of Managers, 1945-55. (Typewritten.)

VIII

Public Documents

58. *Form of citations.*—The form used for citing public documents should be one that makes them readily accessible to anyone wishing to locate them in a library. The arrangement of information on the title pages of the documents themselves, its amount and complexity, raise puzzling questions of how much of the information it is necessary to include and in what order it should be set down in the footnote. Here reference to the card catalogue of the library can be of great help, although it is not a safe guide in such matters as capitalization and punctuation, which for public documents as well as for other references must follow the scheme of the paper. When in doubt of how much to include in a reference, it is better to err on the side of giving too much rather than too little information.

The name of the country, state, city, town, or other government district (e.g., U.S., Great Britain, Illinois, Baltimore) is given first in the citation of an official publication issued by one of them or under its auspices. Then comes the name of the legislative body, court, executive department, bureau, board, commission, or committee. The name of the office rather than the title of the officer should be given except where the title of the officer is the only name of the office, as, for example, "Illinois, State Entomologist." The name of the division, regional office, etc., if any, follows the name of the department, bureau, or commission. Thus the "author" of a document might read: U.S., Department of Labor, Manpower Administration, Office of Manpower Policy, Evaluation, and Research. Following the name of the author, the title of the document, if any, should be given. From this point, the information noted is dependent largely upon the nature of the material.

59. *United States government documents.*—The United States government publishes its official documents in two main categories—the Congressional and the executive departmental.

a) *Congressional documents.*—These include all the documents originating in the Congress. The proceedings of each house, together with the presidential messages, are published in the *Journal*, separately for House and Senate, at the close of each session. The debates appear in the *Congressional Record* (since 1873). Besides the bills and resolutions initiated by the Congress, there are the materials furnished to it by committees, governmental agencies, and executive officers of government—reports, hearings, miscellaneous documents. Citations to all of them must include, in addition to the authorizing body, the number, session, and date of the Congress; title and number (if any) of the document; and, in some instances the title of the work in which the document can be found, with relevant volume and page number(s).

The letters "N." and "B." stand, respectively, for footnote entry and bibliographic entry.

N. [1]U.S., Congress, House, <u>A Bill To Require Passenger-Carrying Motor Vehicles Purchased for Use by the Federal Government To Meet Certain Safety Standards</u>, H.R. 1341, 86th Cong., 1st sess., 1959, pp. 1-3.

B. U.S. Congress. House. <u>A Bill To Require Passenger-Carrying Motor Vehicles Purchased for Use by the Federal Government To Meet Certain Safety Standards</u>. H.R. 1341, 86th Cong., 1st sess., 1959.

N.   [2]U.S., Congress, Senate, <u>Planning in Metropolitan</u>
<u>Areas</u>, S. Rept. 821 To Accompany S. 855, 88th Cong., 2d
sess., 1964, pp. 3, 7.

B.   U.S.   Congress.   Senate.   <u>Planning in Metropolitan Areas</u>.
           S. Rept. 821 To Accompany S. 855, 88th Cong.,
           2d sess., 1964.

N.   [3]U.S., Congress, Senate, <u>Report of the Federal Trade</u>
<u>Commission</u>, S. Doc. 92, 70th Cong., 1st sess., 1935,
pt. 71A.

B.   U.S.   Congress.   Senate.   <u>Report of the Federal Trade Com-</u>
           <u>mission</u>.   S. Doc. 92, 70th Cong., 1st sess., 1935.

N.   [4]U.S., Congress, Senate, Committee on Foreign Relations, <u>Technical Assistance and Related Programs</u>, S. Rept.
1956, 84th Cong., 2d sess., 1960, <u>Senate Miscellaneous</u>
<u>Reports on Public Bills</u>, III, 184-85.

B.   U.S.   Congress.   Senate.   Committee on Foreign Relations.
           <u>Technical Assistance and Related Programs</u>.   S. Rept.
           1956, 84th Cong., 2d sess., 1960.   <u>Senate Miscel-</u>
           <u>laneous Reports on Public Bills</u>, Vol. III.

N.   [5]U.S., Congress, Joint Economic Committee, <u>The Low-</u>
<u>Income Population and Economic Growth</u>, by Robert J. Lampman,
Joint Committee Print, Study Paper 12 (Washington, D.C.:
Government Printing Office, 1959), pp. 14-15.

B.   U.S.   Congress.   Joint Economic Committee.   <u>The Low-Income</u>
           <u>Population and Economic Growth</u>, by Robert J. Lamp-
           man.   Joint Committee Print, Study Paper 12.
           Washington, D.C.: Government Printing Office, 1959.

N.   [6]U.S., Congress, House, <u>The Drug Abuse Control</u>
<u>Amendments of 1965</u>, 89th Cong., 1st sess., 1965, <u>Journal</u>,
March 10, 1965, pp. 337-42.

B.   U.S.   Congress.   House.   <u>The Drug Abuse Control Amendments</u>
           <u>of 1965</u>.   89th Cong., 1st sess., 1965, <u>Journal</u>,
           March 10, 1965.

Hearings should be cited by title, and the particular
House or Senate committee (whether House or Senate committee must be mentioned) before whom the hearings were
held must be included.

N.   [7]U.S., Congress, House, Committee on Ways and Means,
    Narcotics, Marihuana, and Barbiturates, Hearings, before a
    subcommittee of the Committee on Ways and Means, House of
    Representatives, on H.R. 3490, 82d Cong., 1st sess., 1951,
    pp. 2-4.

B.   U.S. Congress. House. Committee on Ways and Means.
         Narcotics, Marihuana, and Barbiturates. Hearings
         before a subcommittee of the Committee on Ways and
         Means, House of Representatives, on H.R. 3490,
         82d Cong., 1st sess., 1951.

Congressional bills and resolutions are published in pamphlet form. When a bill is enacted into law, it becomes a part of the *Statutes at Large*. In the interim between its having been introduced into one of the houses and its passage and publication as a law in the *Statutes*, a bill is cited to the form of the slip bill, or to the *Congressional Record*, if it is contained therein.

N.   [8]U.S., Congress, House, An Act To Amend the Bank
    Holding Company Act of 1956, Pub. L. 89-485, 89th Cong.,
    2d sess., 1966, H.R. 7371, p. 3.

B.   U.S. Congress. House. An Act To Amend the Bank Holding
         Company Act of 1956. Pub. L. 89-485, 89th Cong.,
         2d sess., H.R. 7371.

Congressional debates are printed in the *Congressional Record*. Unless the matter of the speech, or sometimes merely remarks, is mentioned in the text, it is proper to include it in the citation.

N.   [9]U.S., Congress, Senate, Senator Blank speaking for
    the Amendment of the Standing Rules of the Senate, S. Res.
    103, 89th Cong., 1st sess., Nov. 14, 1965, Congressional
    Record, CII, 6522. [A reference to the bound volume, which
    is differently paged from the Daily Digest.]

B.   U.S. Congress. Senate. Senator Blank speaking for the
         Amendment of the Standing Rules of the Senate.
         S. Res. 103, 89th Cong., 1st sess., Nov. 14, 1965.
         Congressional Record, CII, 6522.

Presidential proclamations, executive orders of general interest, and any other documents that the president submits

or orders to be published are carried in the *Federal Register*,
issued on every day following a government working day.

N.   [10]U.S., President, Proclamation, "Supplemental Quota
on Imports of Long-Staple Cotton," Federal Register, XV,
No. 196, Oct. 10, 1950, 6801-6802.

B.   U.S. President. Proclamation. "Supplemental Quota on Im-
       ports of Long-Staple Cotton." Federal Register, XV,
       No. 196, Oct. 10, 1950, 6801-6802.

The papers of the presidents of the United States are collected in two large works that are often cited by students.

N.   [11]J. D. Richardson, ed., Compilation of the Messages
and Papers of the Presidents, 1789-1897 (10 vols. 53d
Cong., 2nd Sess., House Misc. Doc. No. 210, Pts. 1-10
[Washington, D.C.: Government Printing Office, 1907]),
IV, 16.

B.   Richardson, J. D., ed. Compilation of the Messages and
       Papers of the Presidents, 1789-1897. 10 vols. (53d
       Cong., 2d Sess., House Misc. Doc. No. 210, Pts.
       1-10). Washington, D.C.: Government Printing
       Office, 1907.

N.   [12]U.S., President, Public Papers of the Presidents
of the United States (Washington, D.C.: Office of the Federal Register, National Archives and Records Service,
1953-), Dwight D. Eisenhower, 1956, pp. 221-23.

B.   U.S. President. Public Papers of the Presidents of the
       United States. Washington, D.C.: Office of the
       Federal Register, National Archives and Records
       Service, 1953-. Dwight D. Eisenhower, 1956.

After their passage, bills and joint and concurrent resolutions are cited as statutes. Those that have gone into effect
during the year are published in the *Statutes at Large* (n.
13), which since 1939 have been issued annually at the
close of the calendar year. Later, the statutes are published
in the *United States Code. Code* citation is preferred when
it is available (n. 14). As a matter of convenience to the

reader, a statute is sometimes given a parallel citation to the *Statutes at Large* (n. 15).

N.   [13]Administrative Procedure Act, Statutes at Large, LX, sec. 10, 243 (1946).

B.   Administrative Procedure Act. Statutes at Large, Vol. LX (1946).

N.   [14]Declaratory Judgment Act, U.S. Code, Vol. XXVIII, secs. 2201-2202 (1952). [Citations to the Code are always by section number, not page.]

B.   Declaratory Judgment Act. U.S. Code, Vol. XXVIII (1952).

N.   [15]Labor Management Relations Act (Taft-Hartley Act), Statutes at Large, LXI, sec. 301(a), 156 (1947), U.S. Code, Vol. XXXIX, sec. 185(a) (1952).

B.   Labor Management Relations Act (Taft-Hartley Act). Statutes at Large, Vol. LXI (1947). U.S. Code, Vol. XXXIX (1952).

The United States Constitution is referred to by article and section (by clause as well, if relevant). If the reference is to an amendment, it must be cited by number following *"Constitution."*

N.   [16]U.S., Constitution, Art. I, sec. 4.

B.   U.S. Constitution, Art. I, sec. 4.

N.   [17]U.S., Constitution, Amendment XIV, sec. 2.

B.   U.S. Constitution, Amendment XIV, sec. 2.

The several government commissions, such as the Federal Communications Commission, Federal Trade Commission, Securities and Exchange Commission, also publish bulletins, circulars, reports, study papers, and the like. Frequently those communications are classified as House or Senate documents.

N.   [18]U.S., Congress, Senate, <u>Report of the Federal</u>
<u>Trade Commission on Utility Corporations</u>, Sen. Doc. 92, 70th
Cong., 1st sess., 1935, pt. 71 A.

B.   U.S. Congress. Senate. <u>Report of the Federal Trade Commis-</u>
<u>sion on Utility Corporations</u>. Sen. Doc. 92, 70th
Cong., 1st sess., 1935.

b) *Executive departmental documents.*—These consist of reports of executive departments and bureaus, bulletins, circulars, and miscellaneous materials. Many departmental publications are classified in series, and some have personal
authors, whose names are included in the citations (n. 2).
It is not desirable, however, to cite government publications
by names of personal authors. Few libraries catalogue them
except under the names of the sponsoring government
agency.

N.   [1]U.S., Department of Health, Education, and Welfare,
<u>Proceedings, 1961 Conference of the Surgeon-General, Public</u>
<u>Health Service, and Chief, Children's Bureau, with State and</u>
<u>Territorial Health Officers, Aug. 8-10, 1961</u> (Washington,
D.C.: Government Printing Office, 1961), pp. 8-10.

B.   U.S. Department of Health, Education, and Welfare. <u>Proceed-</u>
<u>ings, 1961 Conference of the Surgeon-General, Public</u>
<u>Health Service, and Chief, Children's Bureau, with</u>
<u>State and Territorial Health Officers, Aug. 8-10,</u>
<u>1961.</u> Washington, DC.: Government Printing Office,
1961.

N.   [2]U.S., Department of Agriculture, Farm Security Administration and Bureau of Agricultural Economics Co-operat-
ing, <u>Analysis of 70,000 Rural Rehabilitation Farmlands</u>, by
E. L. Kirkpatrick, Social Research Report No. 9 (Washington,
D.C.: Government Printing Office, 1938), pp. 19-32.

B.   U.S. Department of Agriculture. Farm Security Administration and Bureau of Agricultural Economics Co-operat-
ing. <u>Analysis of 70,000 Rural Rehabilitation Farm-</u>
<u>lands</u>, by E. L. Kirkpatrick. Social Research
Report No. 9. Washington, D.C.: Government Printing Office, 1938.

N.   [3]U.S., Department of State, <u>Declaration of the U.N.</u>
<u>Conference on Food and Agriculture</u>, War Documents Series
Pubn. No. 2162 (1944), pp. 6-8.

B.   U.S. Department of State. <u>Declaration of the U.N. Confer-</u>
              <u>ence on Food and Agriculture.</u> War Documents Series
              Pubn. No. 2162 (1944).

N.   [4]U.S., Department of State, <u>Public Roads Program in</u>
<u>the Philippines</u>, Treaties and Other International Acts Se-
ries 1584, Pubn. 2805 (1947), p. 3. [The number 1584 is the
number of the "treaty" as assigned by the State Department.]

B.   U.S. Department of State. <u>Public Roads Program in the Phil-</u>
              <u>ippines.</u> Treaties and Other International Acts Se-
              ries 1584, Pubn. 2805 (1947).

N.   [5]U.S., Department of Interior, Office of Indian Affairs, <u>Annual Report of the Commissioner of Indian Affairs</u>
<u>to the Secretary of the Interior, for the Fiscal Year ended</u>
<u>June 30, 1932</u> (Washington, D.C.: Government Printing Of-
fice, 1932), p. 24.

B.   U.S. Department of Interior. Office of Indian Affairs. <u>An-</u>
              <u>nual Report of the Commissioner of Indian Affairs to</u>
              <u>the Secretary of the Interior, for the Fiscal Year</u>
              <u>Ended June 30, 1932.</u> Washington, D.C.: Government
              Printing Office, 1932.

N.   [6]U.S., Department of Commerce, Bureau of the Census,
<u>Fifteenth Census of the United States, 1930: Population,</u>
II, 98.

B.   U.S. Department of Commerce. Bureau of the Census. <u>Fif-</u>
              <u>teenth Census of the United States, 1930: Popula-</u>
              <u>tion</u>. Vol. II.

N.   [7]U.S., Department of Commerce, Bureau of the Census,
<u>United States Census of Population: 1960</u>, Vol. I, <u>Charac-</u>
<u>teristics of the Population</u>, pt. 6, California.

B.   U.S. Department of Commerce. Bureau of the Census. <u>United</u>
              <u>States Census of Population: 1960.</u> Vol. I, <u>Charac-</u>
              <u>teristics of the Population</u>, pt. 6, California.

Since 1950, treaties have been published in the series
United States Treaties and Other International Agreements
(n. 8), which is the annual bound volume of the papers as
they were numbered and published by the Department of
State in pamphlet form in the series *Treaties and Other In-*

ternational Acts (n. 4, p. 89). With the inauguration of the new series, publication was discontinued in the *Statutes at Large*. Multilateral treaties appear in the Treaty Series of the United Nations (n. 10), although usually a year or more after their signature. Treaties predating 1950 may be found (depending upon their nature and date) in the Treaty Series of the League of Nations; the Treaty Series and Executive Agreement Series of the Department of State; and in the *Statutes at Large* (n. 9).

N.   [8]U.S., Department of State, <u>United States Treaties and Other International Agreements</u>, Vol. XIV, pt. 2. "Nuclear Weapons Test Ban," TIAS No. 5433, Aug. 5, 1963, pp. 1315-26. [TIAS 5433 refers to the treaty number assigned by the Dept. of State in the <u>Treaties and Other International Acts Series</u>.]

B.   U.S. Department of State. <u>United States Treaties and Other International Agreements</u>, Vol. XIV, pt. 2. "Nuclear Weapons Test Ban," TIAS No. 5433, Aug. 5, 1963.

N.   [9]U.S., <u>Statutes at Large</u>, Vol. XLIII, pt. 2 (Dec. 1923-March 1925), "Naval Armament Limitation Treaty," Feb. 26, 1922, ch. 1, art. 2, p. 1657.

B.   U.S. <u>Statutes at Large</u>, Vol. XLIII, pt. 2 (Dec. 1923-March 1925). "Naval Armament Limitation Treaty," Feb. 26, 1922.

N.   [10]United Nations, Treaty Series, <u>Treaties and International Agreements Registered or Filed and Reported with the Secretariat of the United Nations</u>, Vol. CCL (1956), No. 3516, "Denmark and Italy: Convention Concerning Military Service," July 15, 1954, p. 45.

B.   United Nations. Treaty Series. <u>Treaties and International Agreements Registered or Filed and Reported with the Secretariat of the United Nations</u>, Vol. CCL (1956). No. 3516, "Denmark and Italy: Convention Concerning Military Service," July 15, 1954.

60. *State and local government documents.*—Citations are in essentially the same form as United States government documents.

N.   [1]Illinois, Constitution (1848), art. 5, sec. 2.
[The date of a constitution is indicated ordinarily only
when it is not the one in force.]

B.   Illinois. Constitution (1848).

N.   [2]Kentucky, Revised Statutes, Annotated (Baldwin,
1943). [Refers to an annotated revision made by William E.
Baldwin in 1943.]

B.   Kentucky. Revised Statutes, Annotated (Baldwin, 1943).

N.   [3]Ohio, Judicial Organization Act, Statutes (1830),
III, 1671-78.

B.   Ohio. Judicial Organization Act. Statutes (1830), Vol.
III.

N.   [4]New York, N.Y., "Good Samaritan" Law, Administrative Code (1965), sec. 67-3.2.

B.   New York, N.Y. "Good Samaritan" Law, Administrative Code
(1965).

61. *British government documents.*—Citations to British government documents, like their counterparts in United States documents, should begin with the authority under which they were
issued—Parliament, Public Record Office, Foreign Office, Min-
istry of Transport, and so on, always preceded by "Great
Britain."

English statutes are always cited by name, regnal year of the
sovereign, and chapter number. Names of sovereigns are abbreviated and Arabic numerals are used throughout. Before
publication in the *Statutes* or in the *Public General Acts and
Church Assembly Measures*, statutes are cited as in note 1;
when they are published in one or the other compilations, their
citations follow the forms of notes 2 and 3.

N.   [1]Great Britain, Laws, Statutes, etc., <u>Coroner's Act,</u>
      <u>1954</u>, 2 & 3 Eliz. 2, ch. 31.

B.   Great Britain. <u>Coroner's Act, 1954</u>. 2 & 3 Eliz. 2, ch 31.

N.   [2]Great Britain, Laws, Statutes, etc., <u>Transport Act,</u>
      <u>1962</u>, 10 & 11 Eliz. 2, ch. 46, <u>Halsbury's Statutes of Eng-</u>
      <u>land</u> (2d ed.), XLII, 565-68 (pt. 1, sec. 3-6).

B.   Great Britain. <u>Transport Act, 1962.</u> 10 & 11 Eliz. 2, ch.
           46. <u>Halsbury's Statutes of England</u> (2d ed.), Vol.
           XLII.

N.   [3]Great Britain, Laws, Statutes, etc., <u>Trustee Sav-</u>
      <u>ings Banks Act, 1964</u>, 12 Eliz. 2, ch. 4, <u>The Public General</u>
      <u>Acts and Church Assembly Measures, 1964</u>, pt. 1, p. 6 (sec.
      2/3).

B.   Great Britain. <u>Trustee Savings Banks Act, 1964.</u> 12 Eliz.
           2, ch. 4. <u>The Public General Acts and Church As-</u>
           <u>sembly Measures, 1964</u>, pt. 1.

The *Parliamentary Papers* are bound annually in consecutive volumes of *Bills*, *Reports*, and *Accounts and Papers*. Each of these has its own series of volume numbers, which means that any one title is, for example, volume 2 in its own series and Volume X of the whole *Parliamentary Papers* for the year. In the volumes of *Reports*, the separate individually paged documents are arranged alphabetically by their subjects. Some are "command" papers and are cited as such (n. 4), with number and title if desired.

N.   [4]Great Britain, Parliament, <u>Parliamentary Papers</u>
      (House of Commons & Command), 1962-63, Vol. XIX (<u>Reports</u>,
      vol. 8), Cmnd. 2062, Dec., 1962, "Report of the Ministry of
      Health for the Year Ended 31 December, 1962," ch. ii, pp.
      8-10 [of the report].

B.   Great Britain. Parliament. <u>Parliamentary Papers</u> (House of
           Commons & Command), 1962-63, Vol. XIX (<u>Reports</u>, vol.
           8). Cmnd. 2062. [The title of the report may be
           omitted; the command number identifies it.]

The *Sessional Papers*, which are not to be confused with the *Parliamentary Papers*—which are also sometimes called *Ses-*

sional Papers—have been published since 1938-39 following each session of Parliament, and are separate for the two houses. The series is divided into eight titles—five for the Commons and three for the House of Lords. The annual series of *Papers* is identified by year-date alone, but each of the eight titles has its individual set of volume numbers. A citation to these *Sessional Papers* can be deceiving, since some of the volumes are made up of separate papers that are individually paged and arranged either chronologically by day or alphabetically by subject. Citations should be made, not to page numbers, but to the specific document by its title, with pertinent numbered sections or paragraphs if the paper is long. The books have well-arranged tables of contents and indexes, and locating a particular paper is no problem. (See nn. 5 and 6.)

N.   [5]Great Britain, Parliament, Sessional Papers (House of Commons), 1962-63, Votes and Proceedings: 19 March, 1963,"Navy Supplementary Estimate, 1962-63" (Supply). [No volume number; there was only one in 1962-63. The arrangement is alphabetical by subject--in this case "Supply."]

B.   Great Britain. Parliament. Sessional Papers (House of Commons), 1962-63. Votes and Proceedings: 19 March, 1963, "Navy Supplementary Estimate, 1962-63" (Supply).

N.   [6]Great Britain, Parliament, Sessional Papers (House of Lords), 1962-63, Public Bills, Vol. I: "Contracts of Employment," sec. 2.

B.   Great Britain. Parliament. Sessional Papers (House of Lords), 1962-63. Public Bills, Vol. I: "Contracts of Employment."

Since 1909 the *Parliamentary Debates* have been published separately for the two houses. The name "Hansard" is properly omitted from the title of volumes issued since 1891, but it still has official sanction and is sometimes used even now (n. 8). Both series and volume numbers are required. And since the *Debates* have now passed the 720th volume number, the general rule of expressing volume numbers with Roman numerals is here disregarded and Arabic numerals used in this case (nn. 7, 8).

N.   [7]Great Britain, Parliament, Parliamentary Debates (House of Commons), 5th ser., Vol. 721 (22 Nov.-3 Dec., 1965), pp. 779-87.

B.   Great Britain. Parliament. Parliamentary Debates (House of Commons), 5th ser., Vol. 721 (22 Nov.-3 Dec., 1965).

N.   [8]Great Britain, Parliament, Hansard's Parliamentary Debates, 3d ser., Vol. 30 (1835), p. 452.

B.   Great Britain. Parliament. Hansard's Parliamentary Debates, 3d ser., Vol. 30 (1835).

The *British and Foreign State Papers* are arranged within the volumes alphabetically by country and, further, by subject.

N.   [9]Great Britain, Foreign Office, British and Foreign State Papers, 1852-53, Vol. XLI, "Austria: Proclamation of the Emperor Annulling the Constitution of 4th of March, 1849," pp. 1298-99.

B.   Great Britain. Foreign Office. British and Foreign State Papers, 1852-53, Vol. XLI. "Austria: Proclamation of the Emperor Annulling the Constitution of 4th March, 1849."

Reports are issued in pamphlet form by the several ministries, committees, commissions, and the like.

N.   [10]Great Britain, Office of the Minister of Science, Committee on Management and Control of Research, Report, 1961 (London: Her Majesty's Stationery Office, 1961), p. 58.

B.   Great Britain. Office of the Minister of Science. Committee on Management and Control of Research. Report, 1961. London: Her Majesty's Stationery Office, 1961.

The early records entitled *Calendar of* . . . are arranged chronologically. In some of them numbered items—grants, leases, pardons, warrants, and so on—appear within a "calendar" of no uniform duration (n. 11). Dates are essential, therefore, in identifying the items.

N.   [11]Great Britain, Public Record Office, Calendar of
the Patent Rolls, Elizabeth [1], Vol. IV (1566-69): Calendar 66 (17 Nov. 1566-16 Nov. 1567), 2 May, 1567, No. 455,
Pardon for Richard Byngham, pp. 63-64.

B.   Great Britain. Public Record Office. Calendar of the Pat-
        ent Rolls, Elizabeth [1], Vol. IV (1566-69), Calen-
        dar 66: 2 May, 1567, No. 455.

N.   [12]Great Britain, Public Record Office, Calendar of
State Papers, Domestic, of the Reign of Charles 2, Vol. CCIX
(1667): 12 July, 1667, Earl of Carlisle to Williamson, p.
289.

B.   Great Britain. Public Record Office. Calendar of State
        Papers, Domestic, of the Reign of Charles 2, Vol.
        CCIX (1667): 12 July, 1667, Earl of Carlisle to
        Williamson.

N.   [13]Great Britain, Public Record Office, Calendar of
Treasury Books, Vol. XXXII (1718), pt. 2: 27 February,
"Royal Warrant to the Clerk of the Signet . . ."

B.   Great Britain. Public Record Office. Calendar of Treasury
        Books, Vol. XXXII (1718), pt. 2: 27 February,
        "Royal Warrant to the Clerk of the Signet . . ."

N.   [14]Great Britain, Public Record Office, List and
Analysis of State Papers, Foreign Series, Elizabeth [1]
(1 Aug., 1589-30 June, 1590), Vol. I: III, Spain, No. 637,
"Spanish Agents in England."

B.   Great Britain. Public Record Office. List and Analysis of
        State Papers, Foreign Series. Elizabeth [1] (1
        August, 1589-30 June, 1590), Vol. I: III, Spain,
        No. 637.

62. *League of Nations and United Nations documents.*—Besides the
authorizing body, the topic of the paper with document number
and date must be given.

N.   [1]League of Nations, Secretariat, <u>Application of Part
II of the Opium Convention</u> (O.C. 114) (1923), p. 5.

B.   League of Nations. Secretariat. <u>Application of Part II of
      the Opium Convention</u> (O.C. 114) (1923).

N.   [2]United Nations, Economic and Social Council, Social
Commission, 17th Session, <u>Reappropriation of the Role of the
Social Commission: Report of the Secretary-General</u> (E/CN.
5/400), Feb. 16, 1966, pp. 9-10.

B.   United Nations. Economic and Social Council. Social Com-
            mission, 17th Session. <u>Reappropriation of the Role
            of the Social Commission: Report of the Secretary
            General</u> (E/CN.5/400), February 16, 1966.

N.   [3]United Nations, General Assembly, 17th Session,
Oct. 8, 1966, <u>Report of the Special Committee on the Situa-
tion with regard to the Implementation of the Declaration on
the Granting of Independence to Colonial Countries and Peo-
ples</u>, A/5238, Annex 1, p. 3.

B.   United Nations. General Assembly, 17th Session, October 8,
            1966. <u>Report of the Special Committee on the Situa-
            tion with regard to the Implementation of the Decla-
            ration on the Granting of Independence to Colonial
            Countries and Peoples</u>, A/5238.

N.   [4]United Nations, World Health Organization, <u>Toxic
Hazards of Pesticides to Man: Twelfth Report of the Expert
Committee on Insecticides</u> (WHO Technical Report Series, No.
227), 1962, pp. 6-10.

B.   United Nations. World Health Organization. <u>Toxic Hazards
            of Pesticides to Man: Twelfth Report of the Expert
            Committee on Insecticides</u>. WHO Technical Report Se-
            ries, No. 227, 1962.

IX

Scientific Papers

63. It is difficult to generalize about the format of scientific papers as distinct from other kinds of scholarly papers, not only because practice varies somewhat from field to field, but also because even within the same field variable factors determine style to some extent. In general, however, there are three major differences between format in non-scientific and in scientific papers: (1) organization, (2) handling of references, and (3) use of numerals, symbols, and abbreviations.

In such mechanical matters as spacing and pagination, and the presentation of tables and other illustrative materials, the scientific paper should conform in general to the style recommended in this manual under the several headings.

64. *Organization.*—The length of the paper determines quite largely whether it is typed continuously, that is, without beginning new pages for each major section, as is common in most short papers; whether each major section begins on a new page, without, however, formally designating each section as chapter or part; or whether each section, designated as chapter or part, begins on a new page, as is generally the practice in a long paper.

In the first two types, the major divisions may or may not be both numbered and titled, but properly they should be marked by either number or title. In all three types subheadings usually appear within the major divisions, but, in general, these should not begin new pages. (Suitable styles of subheadings and some suggestions on their logical order are discussed in sec. 10, pp. 5-6).

In short papers it is not necessary to include a table of contents, a list of tables, or a list of illustrations, although individual preferences or the demands of a specific piece of writing may call for one or all of these.

65. *References.*—In papers in scientific fields, the general practice is to collect all the references at the end of the paper under some such heading as "List of References" or "Literature Cited." The term "Bibliography" appears less often, since for the most part it is not appropriate, the "List" usually being confined to those works mentioned in the paper. But if the list actually is a bibliography, it should be so headed.

Under the list scheme—regardless of its heading—one of two styles of reference index in the text is used most often.

a) The surname of the author with year-date of the publication enclosed in parentheses; or year-date alone if the author's name occurs in the sentence. The list of references is arranged alphabetically by surnames of authors. When there are two or more works by the same author, they are listed chronologically. Two or more works by the same author published in the same year are identified as, for example, 1964*a*, 1964*b*. Unless a particular purpose is served by numbering the entries in the list, numbering is omitted. Suggested styles of entries are the following:

Article

Mohr, H. 1962. Primary effect of light on growth. <u>Ann. Rev.
Plant Physiol.</u> 13: 465-88. [The first figure is volume
number; figures following the colon are page numbers.]

Book

Kramer, P. J., and Kozlowski, T. T. 1960. <u>Physiology of trees.</u>
P. 11. New York: McGraw-Hill.

If reference to specific parts of a work—page(s), table, illustration—is desired, the notation should be included in the textual reference rather than in the entry in the list. Following are examples of textual references mentioning specific parts:

```
     "Analysis of the paired-data variance (table 2, Goulden,
1952) yields . . . "

     "Ulrich (1927, p. 29 and Fig. 2) divided the Simpson
into . . . "
```

In the foregoing examples of entries in a list of references, the reference to a journal article cites the title of the article, using capitalization as in a sentence. In some fields it is usual to omit the title of the article. The decision to include or to omit the titles must be made before the list is compiled, and one scheme consistently followed. The student may be guided in this decision by observing the general practice of journals in his field. If the paper is to be submitted to a specific journal for publication, it is well to follow exactly the style of reference used by that journal.

b) An Arabic numeral placed between parentheses (sometimes between square brackets []) on the line with the text, following the author's name. The number agrees with the specific reference in the list of references. The references may run in numerical order through the paper, with interruptions in the order when an earlier reference is cited again. If this scheme is used, the list of references cannot be in alphabetical order—an obvious disadvantage. On the other hand, alphabetization requires that the list be compiled in advance. Numerical sequence of references in the text is thus impossible, but a greater disadvantage lies in the difficulty of making changes in the list once it is compiled and numbers assigned to the entries. Scheme *a*, far less susceptible to error, should be preferred to *b*.

Under either scheme, standard abbreviations for the names of journals are recommended. A list is available in *Chemical Abstracts List of Periodicals* (Washington, D.C.: American Chemical Society, 1961). If the names of publishers are given in shortened form, as is recommended, standard abbreviations should be used in accordance with the list given in *Books in Print,* published annually by R. R. Bowker Co., New York, or, for British publishers, in the *Reference Catalogue of Current Literature,* Volume I, published annually by J. Whitaker & Sons, London.

66. *Footnotes.*—Although the practice of collecting references in a list at the end of the paper appears to be growing in use, it is by no means uniform even within a given field, and the citing of references in footnotes is not uncommon. They follow the same general pattern of an entry in a list of references except that the author's name is usually given in normal order—Mark E. Jones, not Jones, Mark E. The reference index is ordinarily a superscript numeral, agreeing with the numeral identifying the footnote. The numerals may begin with "1" on each page, or they may run consecutively through the paper.

Relevant material not of sufficient importance to be brought into the text of the paper may be put into footnotes. It should not be placed in the list of references. When the scheme adopted is to put the references to the literature into footnotes, content footnotes should be numbered consecutively with the reference footnotes. When the scheme is to put all the references to the literature into a list at the end of the paper, the content footnotes should be numbered separately, beginning with "1" and numbering them consecutively through the entire paper. To distinguish them clearly from the references to the literature, these content footnotes should be indicated by superscript Arabic numerals.

67. *Styles of reference.*—The following examples are for entries in a list of references in some cases and for footnotes in others. They are patterned after the styles used by the leading publications in the several fields.

a) *Anthropology.*—There is some variation in practice within this field. The scheme of the *American Anthropologist* is shown here. References to the literature are given in the text of the paper. The author's surname (unless it occurs in the text), year-date of the publication, and page number are enclosed in parentheses: "(Herskovits, 1952: 12)." An alphabetized bibliography at the end of the paper supplies complete information in the following forms:

Journal reference

KLUCKHOHN, C.
1943   Covert culture and administrative problems.
              American Anthropologist 45: 213-227.

Book reference

SCHALLER, G. B.
1963   The mountain gorilla. Chicago, University of
              Chicago Press.

b) *Chemistry.*—Uses footnote references, each bearing a number.

Journal reference

(10) W. G. Lloyd and C. E. Lange, J. Am. Chem. Soc., 86, 1491
     (1964).

Book reference

(18) J. S. Rowlinson, "Liquids and Liquid Mixtures," Butterworth
     and Co., Ltd., London, 1959, p. 14.

c) *Mathematics.*—Uses an alphabetized list of references, each entry being numbered.

Journal reference

7. Hans Samelson, Topology of Lie groups, Bull. Amer. Math.
     Soc. 58 (1952), 2-37.

Book reference

9. G. N. Watson, A treatise on the theory of Bessel functions,
     2d ed., Cambridge, 1962, p. 11.

d) *Physics.*—Uses footnote references.

Journal reference
[1]P. G. Burke and K. Smith, Rev. Mod. Phys. 34, 458 (1962).

Book reference
[4]H. A. Bethe, Intermediate Quantum Mechanics (W. Benjamin, Inc.,
New York, 1964), pp. 29-30.

e) *Psychology.*—Uses footnote references.

Journal reference
[1]R. A. McCleary, Type of response as a factor in interocular
transfer in fish, J. Comp. Physiol. Psychol., 53, 1960, 311-32.

Book reference
[9]R. S. Woodworth and Harold Schlosberg, Exper. Psychol. (2d
ed.), 1954, 200.

68. *Numerals, symbols, and abbreviations.*—The demand in scientific papers for the use of numbers and units of measurement expressed in numerical values makes it suitable for purposes of clarity to use figures, symbols, and abbreviations to an extent not considered good form in non-scientific writing. Aside from a few rules here set down, the writer must settle on the scheme he will use—preferably when working on his first draft—and maintain the same usage throughout the paper.

a) Spell out a number at the beginning of a sentence, even if it is part of a connected group for which numerals are used after it. A better plan in such circumstances is to reconstruct the sentence so as not to begin with a number.

b) Spell out expressions of measurement when they are not preceded by numbers.

c) To avoid confusion, spell out one set of figures in an expression involving two or more series of figures.

> In a test given six months later, ninety-seven children made no errors; eighty-two made 1-2 errors; sixty-four made 3-4 errors.

d) Do not use the symbol for *per cent* (%) when it is not preceded by a figure. *Percentage,* not *per cent* or %, is the correct expression to use when no figure is given.

> The September scores showed an improvement of 70.1% [or 70.1 per cent if the writer prefers to spell out]. Thus the percentage of achievers in the second test indicated . . .

In mathematical text the demands for the use of symbols and abbreviations are so complicated, and vary so much from one paper to another, that no suggestions can be given here. Students in this field should receive training in correct usage along with their education in the science. Editors of some of the mathematical periodicals have prepared manuals for authors which give useful suggestions.

X

Tables

69. If tables are to serve satisfactorily the purpose for which they are made, they not only must be accurately compiled but must be so arranged that they can be easily read and interpreted. To these ends careful spacing, lining, arrangement of headings, period leaders, and, finally, the placing of the tables with respect to the text all contribute.

70. *Placement.*—Ideally, a table should follow immediately after it is first mentioned in the text. But this is not always possible if other matters equally as important as position are considered, as they must be. It is only sensible to expect that tables a page or less in length will be presented in one piece. If, then, the place at which the table is first mentioned is so far down on the page that the table in its entirety cannot be accommodated, the typist may well be puzzled, especially since the general rule is to fill all pages whenever possible. The only answer to the puzzle is to omit the table at the point of its first mention, continue the text following it to the end of the page, and put the table at the top of the next page. As a matter of fact, if space permits, the text should continue at the top of the second page until the end of a paragraph is reached; but this of course must not be done unless there is ample space both to complete the paragraph and to type the entire table.

A table over a page in length should begin immediately after it is first mentioned in the text, since it would have to be divided in any case.

If a table is wider than can be accommodated on one page in regular position and therefore must be placed either the long way of the paper or on facing pages (see Tables 6 and 7), it can be introduced immediately following its first mention only if that mention should come at the bottom of a page. Since this rarely happens, the typing of the text must continue to the foot of the page, and the table be placed on the next page (or pages). The completing of a paragraph on the same page as the table is in this case not permissible, since textual matter should not appear on the same pages with either broadside tables or facing tables.

Tables may be set to occupy the full width of the typed page or, if the columnar matter permits, less than the full width but in any case centered horizontally upon the page.

71. *Long, narrow tables.*—When a table is long and narrow, space may be saved by doubling—dividing it vertically in equal parts and setting them side by side (see Table 2).

72. *Tables more than a page in width.*—Wide tables may be placed broadside (see Table 6). The table number and the caption should be at the binding side of the page. If too wide to be accommodated broadside, a table may be arranged on two facing pages (see Table 7). The parts of the table must be of the same dimensions on both pages, and special care in typing will be required to insure that the appropriate figure in each column is exactly in line with the item in the stub (i.e., first column) to which it belongs.

Tables too wide to be accommodated on the 8½-×-11-inch page in either of the ways described may be typed on two or more pages, which then may be pasted together and reduced to page size by a suitable photographic process; or, less satisfactorily for the use of any paper that is to be bound and placed in a library, a large table may be folded (see sec. 92, p. 124-25).

73. *Continuation of tables more than a page in length.*—Long tables may be continued from page to page. The table number and the caption are typed at the beginning of the table; the table number only on succeeding pages, written, for example, "TABLE 2—Continued." Ordinarily, the box headings above the columns are repeated on every page, except that in a continued *broadside table in which the pages face* the headings need not be repeated on the second page (and the fourth, sixth, etc., if the table is at least four pages).

74. *Table number and caption.*—Center "TABLE 00," in capital letters on a line by itself, with the number in Arabic numerals. Center the caption, also in capital letters, on the second space below the table number. If the caption is longer than the table is wide, set it in two or more lines, arranging in inverted-pyramid form, single-spaced. Single-space before beginning the first rule above the box headings.

If most of the tables in the paper have captions of two or more lines, space will be saved and the appearance of the tables will be improved by typing the captions in a style different from that just described. Type the table number (written "TABLE 00," as above) flush with the left-hand edge of the table, add a period and a dash, and begin the caption, typing the first line the full width of the table, and centering the succeeding lines. Capitalization may be either of the first word and all proper nouns and proper adjectives, or of the first and last word and all nouns, pronouns, adjectives, adverbs, and verbs.

```
TABLE 4.--Precipitin tests on sera of patients with paragonimia-
            sis: starch block-separated antigens
```

One style of caption must be used consistently throughout the paper.

It is not permissible to give captions for some tables and not for others. If a very brief tabulation is introduced in such a way that a caption seems unnecessary, the tabulation should not be given a table number.

75. *Box Headings.*—These may be of a single level or of two or more levels consisting of spanner headings and subsumed headings (see Table 5). Center all headings above the columns to which they belong and leave the same amount of blank space (at least one) above and below the horizontal rules. *Never* place a horizontal rule immediately beneath a heading lest the rule be taken for underlining of the words. To allow for the vertical rules, leave at least one space at either end of the longest line in each heading.

If a description or classification of the line headings in the stub would be difficult to express briefly, leave the box empty or substitute the word "Item."

Box headings may be typed broadside if necessary to conserve space. They should be set so as to read up from the bottom of the page (see Table 6). It will be observed that if a table is typed the long way of the paper and the box headings are then typed vertically, the headings will be upside down when the page is in regular position. This cannot be avoided. Single-space all box headings.

Numbering the headings is a convenience if the textual discussion refers to individual columns. The numbers should be placed in parentheses and centered on the first line below the box headings. The heading above the stub should be numbered "(1)" and the subsequent headings follow in numerical sequence (see Table 3).

76. *Cut-in headings.*—At times the use of cut-in headings, as shown in Table 5 ("Males," "Females"), will permit the combining of data in one table that without them would require two or more tables. Cut-in headings should be centered and capitalized to accord with the scheme used for the box headings.

77. *Stub.*—Runovers in line headings in the stub are indented to the third space unless the heading has subdivisions.

```
Coastal district vs. interior
   district
```

Runovers are indented to the fifth space if the heading is subdivided, the subdivisions being indented to the third space.

```
Relative to issue
    price:
  1923-27 . . . .
  1949-55 . . . .
```

The words "Total," "Mean," and "Average" in the stub should also be indented.

If the open space between the stub and the first column is such that the eye does not travel easily from the line heading to the related figure or word in the column, period leaders (spaced periods) should connect the two (see Table 4).

78. *Capitalization.*—Adapt the capitalization of the box headings, stub, and columnar matter to that of the table caption. That is, if the caption is either in capitals throughout or in capitals for the first and last words and all nouns, pronouns, adjectives, adverbs, and verbs, the box headings preferably should be the latter, and the stub and columnar matter preferably in capitals only for first words, proper nouns, and proper adjectives. But if the table caption employs capitals only for the first word, proper nouns, and proper adjectives, the capitalization of the box headings, stub, and columnar matter preferably should agree with that of the caption.

79. *Omissions in columns.*—In a long column of figures, zero preceding a decimal may be omitted from all entries except the first and the last. Degree and dollar signs must be repeated at the top of each column and after every break of the column, such as rules above totals and cut-in headings. If all the figures are in thousands or in millions, space may be saved by omitting the relevant zeroes in the columns and noting this fact at the end of the caption, for example, "(Figures in Millions)" (see Table 4). A blank space in a column should carry period leaders (see Table 7).

80. *Aligning in columns.*—Align all columns of figures by the decimal points. In columns containing dissimilar items, center the dissimilar items and align the decimal points of figures even though figures may be interspersed with other items (see Table 4). Align plus, minus, and plus-minus signs (see Table 5).

81. *Abbreviations and symbols.*—Although for the most part prohibited in text, abbreviations and symbols are legitimate space-saving devices in box headings and in the main body of tables, but not in the captions. Standard abbreviations should be used if they exist, but the writer may devise abbreviations when they do not. Possibly ambiguous abbreviations should be explained in a note or a key. Symbols that cannot be made with the typewriter should be inserted by hand, using permanent black ink (India preferred). A plus sign made with the hyphen and diagonal ($+$) is *not* an acceptable substitute. The hyphen made with the typewriter, and the vertical bar inserted in ink, is satisfactory.

82. *Footnotes to tables.*—Put all footnotes to tables immediately below the tables, not at the foot of the page with footnotes to the text. Begin the first note on the second space below the bottom rule, indenting the first line of each note, single-spacing within the note, and double-spacing between the individual notes. Because footnote indexes in tables usually follow numerals, small letters ("a," "b," etc.) rather than Arabic numerals should be used. If none of the tables in the paper has more than one footnote, an asterisk may be used instead of "a," but the use of doubled and tripled asterisks, or of an asterisk part of the time and letters part of the time, should be avoided.

83. *Ruling.*—Two-column tables should be left completely unruled (see Table 1). In general, all tables of more than two columns should be ruled throughout. It is permissible, however, to omit the rules *within* a group of columns covered by a spanner heading, provided that the columns are not too close together. In Table 3, for example, omission of a rule between Columns 2 and 3 and between Columns 4 and 5 is allowable. But in Table 5 the columns of figures are so close together that the rules are important for ease in reading, and therefore are not omitted. Put a double rule at the top and a vertical double rule between sections of a table that is doubled (see Table 2). Normally, no other double rules should be used.

As has been said (see sec. 75, p. 107), a blank space should be left on all sides of box headings. It is never permissible to begin a heading on the line immediately below a rule, or to rule immediately under a heading (thus giving the effect of underlining of the words).

The rule above the figures for totals, means, and averages should not be extended through the stub (see Table 3).

In a table continued from page to page, the bottom rule should be omitted on all pages except the last.

Normally, horizontal rules are made with the typewriter; vertical rules, by hand (using permanent black ink, preferably India). If the carriage of the typewriter takes the paper the long way, all the rules may be made with the typewriter. Using the typewriter for the vertical rules will require particular care if the columns are only one or two spaces apart.

Since some institutions specify that all tables shall be ruled and others allow considerable latitude, it is advisable to check into the matter with the appropriate staff officer.

84. *Spacing.*—Reference to the proper spacing for captions, box headings, and footnotes has been made in the individual sections given to those topics. Other rules to be observed are the following: Three spaces should be left above and three spaces below (i.e., typing should begin on the third space below) tables inserted into text. Typing of the main body of the tables may be either single space or double space or space and one-half, and it need not be the same for all the tables.

TABLE 1

MULTIPLE CORRELATION COEFFICIENTS
OF PROBABILITY FUNCTIONS

Range of Values	No. Observed Values
0-.199	15
.2-.399	1
.4-.599	1

TABLE 2

CASES FILED, TERMINATED, AND PENDING IN THE COURT OF APPEALS
FOR THE THIRD CIRCUIT, FISCAL YEARS 1940-1949, INCLUSIVE

Fiscal year	Com-menced	Termi-nated	Pend-ing	Fiscal Year	Com-menced	Termi-nated	Pend-ing
1940	322	360	170	1945	299	268	226
1941	285	350	102	1946	197	274	149
1942	292	222	172	1947	266	216	199
1943	353	302	223	1948	287	250	236
1944	276	304	195	1949 (1st half)	128	113	251

TABLE 3

ADULT OFFSPRING OF 244 ARKANSAS FARM FAMILIES
BY EDUCATION AND PLACE OF RESIDENCE

Schooling (Years)	Living on Farms		Living in Towns	
	Individuals		Individuals	
	Number	Percentage	Number	Percentage
(1)	(2)	(3)	(4)	(5)
8 or less	350	71[a]	211	60[a]
Above 8	142	29	139	40
10 and over	105	21	116	33
12 and over	62	13	72	21
14 and over	9	2	33	9
16 and over	3	1	15	4
Total	492	. .	. .	. .

[a]All differences over 3 times Standard Error.

TABLE 4

ESTIMATED NATIONAL INCOME OF INDIA, AT 1948-49 PRICES
1900-1901 TO 1950-51, BY SELECTED YEARS
(Money Amounts in Millions of Rupees)

	1900-1901	1910-11	1920-21	1930-31	1904-41	1950-51
Total income						
Amount	51,090	62,410	64,690	76,840	86,460	91,920
Index	100.0	122.1	126.6	150.4	169.2	179.9
Agricultural production						
Amount	39,760	44,330	38,070	45,980	45,340	44,050
Index	100.0	111.5	95.7	115.6	114.0	110.8
All other industries						
Amount	11,330	18,080	26,620	30,860	41,120	48,070
Index	100.0	159.6	234.9	272.4	362.9	424.8

Source: V. K. R. V. Rao, A. K. Ghosh, M. V. Divatia, and Uma Datta, eds.,
Papers on National Income and Allied Topics (Indian Conference on
Research in National Income, Vol. II) (Bombay: Asia Publishing
House, 1962), Table 3, pp. 22-23.

TABLE 5

EFFECT OF A SINGLE 24-HOUR EXPOSURE TO 33 DEGREES C. DURING
DIFFERENT PERIODS OF PUPAL DEVELOPMENT,
REMAINDER OF TIME AT 25 DEGREES C.

Period at 33 Degrees	No. Flies Emerged	Time in Days			Percentage of Development					
		Low Temp.	High Temp.	Total	Per day		Low Temp.	High Temp.	Total	Total −100
					Low Temp.	High Temp.				
Males										
First day	61	3.31	1.00	4.31±0.009	23.47	27.54	77.68	27.54	105.22	+5.22
Second day	64	3.27	1.00	4.27±0.009	23.47	27.54	76.74	27.54	104.28	+4.28
Third day	62	3.14	1.00	4.14±0.020	23.47	27.54	73.69	27.54	101.23	+1.23
Fourth day	66	3.00	0.92	3.92±0.005	23.47	27.54	70.41	25.33	95.74	−4.26
Females										
First day	39	3.08	1.00	4.08±0.009	24.87	28.57	76.59	28.57	105.16	+5.16
Second day	53	2.94	1.00	3.94±0.006	24.87	28.57	73.11	28.57	101.68	+1.68
Third day	58	2.82	1.00	3.82±0.011	24.87	28.57	70.13	28.57	98.70	−1.30
Fourth day	51	3.00	0.86	3.66±0.007	24.87	28.57	74.64	24.57	99.21	−0.79

VALUE ADDED BY MANUFACTURER PER PRODUCTION WORKER (IN DOLLARS), SOUTH BEND STANDARD METROPOLITAN AREA AND SEVEN SELECTED STANDARD METROPOLITAN AREAS, 1947[a]

Census Groups and Code Number	South Bend	South Bend Rank among Selected Standard Metropolitan Areas	Chicago	Indianapolis	St. Louis	Detroit	Toledo	Grand Rapids	Milwaukee
20. Food & kindred products	9,183	5	9,340	8,585	8,777	8,296	7,600	7,709	11,932
23. Apparel & related products	3,797	11	5,397	5,017	4,588	5,170	4,495	5,081	4,732
24. Lumber & products, except furniture	5,629	2	5,503	3,700	4,464	7,569	5,124	5,168	5,262
26. Paper & allied products	7,111	6	6,605	7,286	5,781	6,491	6,629	7,858	7,804
27. Printing & publishing industries	9,767	4	9,125	10,040	8,660	11,528	10,350	8,990	7,888
32. Stone, clay & glass products	4,033	11	6,558	6,058	5,663	6,563	10,284	6,049	6,383
33. Primary metal industries	6,397	4	6,689	4,321	5,599	5,600	6,668	5,263	6,453
34. Fabricated metal products	5,351	10	6,534	5,037	5,687	5,569	5,759	5,884	6,928
35. Machinery, except electrical	6,048	10	6,656	5,502	5,756	6,847	7,298	7,022	6,368
36. Electrical machinery	6,613	6	6,682	6,614	6,054	6,862	5,823	. .[b]	6,243
39. Miscellaneous manufactures	4,755	7	6,042	5,521	4,760	5,825	4,608	5,239	4,642

[a]Calculated from: U.S. Department of Commerce, Bureau of the Census, Census of Manufactures: 1947 (Washington: U.S. Government Printing Office), Vol. III, Statistics by States, pp. 205-9, 308-8, 343-50, 479-81, 483, 648-49.

[b]Complete figures are not provided by the Census.

TABLE 7

CASE LOAD PER JUDGESHIP FOR THE NORTHERN DISTRICT OF FLORIDA
FOR THE FISCAL YEARS 1940-1948, INCLUSIVE
(CASES FILED PER JUDGE)

Fiscal Year	Number of Judges, Florida (Northern)	Total Civil Cases per Judge		Criminal Cases per Judge	
		Florida (Northern)	84 Districts	Florida (Northern)	84 Distr
1940	1	95	153	191	178
1941	1	104	164	247	165
1942	1	103	168	147	174
1943	1	79	158	105	190
1944	1	70	169	161	211
1945	1	98	295	239	209
1946	1	131	321	125	171
1947	1	106	271	110	173
1948	1	85	205	206	167

Notes:
　　During the entire period covered by the table there were 3 judges
signed to the southern district of Florida and 1 to the northern district.
all these years except the fiscal year 1948, there was 1 "roving judge" fo
both districts, but as almost all his time was spent in the southern distr
the case load for 1940-48 has been figured on the basis of 1 judge in the
northern district.
　　Because case-load figures are given to the nearest whole number, i
not always possible to derive exact totals by adding component parts.

TABLE 7--<u>Continued</u>

United States Civil Cases per Judge (United States a Party)						Private Civil Cases per Judge, Total	
Total		OPA		Other United States			
Florida (Northern)	84 Districts	Florida (Northern)	84 Districts	Florida (Northern)	84 Districts	Florida (Northern)	84 Districts
61	72	..	..	61	72	34	81
59	83	..	..	59	83	45	82
70	91	..	..	70	91	33	77
49	100	..	12	49	88	30	58
47	113	7	37	40	76	23	56
70	238	6	160	64	78	28	57
03	251	71	174	32	77	28	70
80	162	30	84	50	78	26	109
63	87	6	20	57	67	22	117

XI

Illustrations

85. In addition to tables, illustrative materials may consist of graphs —pies, curves, and map graphs—charts showing organization of departments, plans, and so on, diagrams of machines and instruments, maps, photographs, commercial illustrations, and original illustrations.

It is not within the scope of this manual to give advice on the inclusion of illustrative materials, or on what type or types to use, or, except in general terms, to give instructions on their presentation. These matters are fully treated in a number of specialized books and manuals.[1] Some general principles of preparation and presentation need to be summarized to bring the form of illustrative materials into harmony with that of the text.

86. *Margins.*—A margin of at least one inch (more is permissible) should be allowed on all four sides of a page carrying illustrative material. Descriptive matter, legend or caption—everything but the page numbers—must fall within the margin.

87. *General form of presentation.*—Line graphs and bar charts may be either (1) drawn in India ink on cross-ruled paper of the same, or approximately the same, quality as the paper used

---

[1] One deserves special mention: Frances W. Zweifel, *A Handbook of Biological Illustration*, Phoenix Science Series (Chicago: University of Chicago Press, 1961). Although as the title implies, the emphasis is on biological illustrations, the treatment of many of the topics is equally helpful in other fields.

for the text; (2) drawn first on cross-ruled paper, traced on the plain bond paper, and the lines inked in; or (3) drawn first and then reproduced by a suitable photographic process. Graph paper is available which is ruled either in the metric system or in inches and fractions thereof. Also, the paper is made with lines in one of several colors: black, brown, red, green, violet, blue. The choice of color may depend upon whether the drawing is to be photographed and whether it is desired to show the entire grid system. The pale blue lines will not reproduce in the photographic process.

When fine detail is to be shown in an illustration, it is sometimes advisable, if not necessary, to make the original drawing larger than could be accommodated on $8\frac{1}{2}$-x-11-inch paper. Made to scale, the illustration is then reduced to page size by photography.

Photographs may be finished either in the $8\frac{1}{2}$-x-11-inch size so as to avoid mounting, or smaller and mounted two or more to a page on the regular typing paper. If photographs are finished full size, the paper should be medium weight, since the heavier weight tends to break in binding. Matte-surface photographs should be preferred to glossy prints, although the latter make sharper illustrations and are therefore a better choice where minute detail must be shown.

Commercial illustrations usually require mounting. If several copies of these are needed, and are not available, the originals may be reproduced photographically. If they are in color, however, photographs may not be satisfactory. The inclusion of illustrations in color may require considerable forethought. As a matter of fact, color cannot be used in a thesis or dissertation for a university or college which requires a planographic or microphotographic reproduction of its theses and dissertations. The photographs and photographic reproductions for use in such theses or dissertations should preferably be on glossy paper.

Many kinds of maps are available ready made, and some may serve satisfactorily with no additions except page and figure number and, possibly, a caption. Some may be used as base maps, with crosshatching, outlining of specific areas, spotting, figures or letters superimposed to produce illustrations adequate for the writer's particular purposes. Unless stippling or crosshatching of only a small area is required, handwork should not be attempted. Two commercial products offer satisfactory methods in combination with handwork: (1) drawing in the conventional manner with black waterproof ink on Craftint, a paper with invisible patterns that are brought out by application of a liquid developer to those parts of the drawing where stippling or crosshatching is desired; (2) drawing outlines on the regular typing paper or on a light-weight drawing paper and applying Zip-a-tone to the areas where stippling or crosshatching is desired. Craftint comes in two styles: singletone Craftint offers three patterns of shading, and the doubletone offers four. A thin gummed paper, Zip-a-tone is available in many different patterns and is made in two styles, with the printing either on the adhesive side or on the upper surface. The first is the simpler to apply. The use of either Craftint or Zip-a-tone presupposes photographic reproduction for presentation in the paper.

Maps often need to be executed entirely by hand. In the fields of geography and geology, where knowledge of maps and map making is so important an objective in the student's training, handmade maps in theses and dissertations, at least, are likely to be a requirement.

88. *Handwork.*—Legends, keys, captions, and any necessary lines, letters, or symbols not present in the illustration proper may be made either with the typewriter or by hand, using black waterproof drawing ink. For hand lettering, the aid of a stencil or a lettering device is recommended to assure clear, even, well-spaced lettering. Since the use of color is not always feasible, various styles of lines must be used in graphs employing two or more curves; and crosshatching, shading with dots and smaller circles, or similar devices should be used in bar charts. (See sec. 87 above regarding use of Craftint and Zip-a-tone.)

89. *Legends and captions.*—If a paper contains several types of illustrations such as graphs, charts, maps, diagrams, it is desirable to label them all figures and number consecutively in Arabic numerals. If there is a disproportionately large number of one type, this should be given its own label and numbered in Arabic numerals in a separate series: Map 1, Chart 10, Graph 15. The number and legend may be centered below the illustration in one of the following styles. The first is suitable for a short figure legend; the second, for a long one.

Fig. 1.--Block diagram of Fern Lake

Fig. 4.--Diagram of gross abnormalities observed in guinea pigs approximately 130 days after infection by one of 6 different strains of Br. abortus.

If the margin below the illustration is not deep enough to carry the figure legend and still allow the one inch of free space, the figure number may be typed at the top center or at the right in the open space surrounding the illustration proper. Sometimes illustrations—maps in particular—carry printed or hand-lettered captions at the top or side, in which case the figure number alone should be centered beneath the illustration.

A key or scale of miles, if included, ordinarily should be typed in a convenient open space surrounding the illustration rather than below it.

Normally full-page illustrations—especially photographic representations in light and shadow—should be labeled plates and numbered in capital Roman numerals (e.g., PLATE VI) centered above the illustration.

If a plate is composed of more than one illustration, these may be individually labeled, either with a figure number alone or with both figure number and legend. If there are many figures on the page and each requires a legend, the illustrations may be numbered, and the figure legends either grouped at the foot of the page or placed on the facing page. A page containing several illustrations, each with its figure legend, need not be labeled a plate; but, for easy reference to the group as a whole, the plate number is a convenience.

A plate may carry a title or not. If it does, the title may be centered (in capital letters throughout) either above or below the illustration; the plate number remains at the top. If there is not space for the title and/or the plate number on the page with the illustration, these may be centered on the facing page. Since typing on photographic paper is not satisfactory, the labeling of a full-page illustration on sensitized paper will have to be done on the facing page.

90. *Placement.*—In general, illustrations should follow as closely as possible the first references to them in text. As with tables (see sec. 70, pp. 104-5), these preferred positions are not always possible, and in some papers there may be sound reasons for grouping all the illustrations, if they are of one type, at the end. If there is a frontispiece, it should face the title page.

Either singly or in groups, illustrations may be placed the long way of the paper if this arrangement is better suited to their proportions. The appropriate label (plate number and title, or figure legend) should be typed broadside, so as to appear directly above or below the illustration, as may be suitable for its type. The top of the illustration should be at the binding side, and the page number should occupy its normal position.

91. *Mounting.*—Illustrations smaller than 8½ x 11 inches must be mounted on bond typing paper. Dry mounting tissue is the most satisfactory adhesive for the purpose. Properly applied—and correct application is most important—the mounts will remain firm for many years without causing the slightest deterioration of the illustrations. The tissue is available in sheets or in rolls, accompanied with complete directions for its use, and can be purchased from any photographic supply store.

Although dry mounting tissue is the preferred adhesive for mountings designed to withstand use for many years, white casein glue is a reasonably satisfactory substitute, provided that it is applied in such a way that buckling does not result. The secret is in using a small enough quantity of the glue so that the liquid does not penetrate the body of the typing paper and cause it to stretch and wrinkle. It would be well to experiment a bit before doing the final mountings. For small mounts, apply the glue thinly just within the edges of the mount. In addition, for larger pieces to be mounted, small dabs of glue applied here and there over the surface may be more satisfactory than its application at the edges alone. Notice that the adhesive is to be applied to the material that is to be mounted, not to the paper beneath it.

The use of rubber cement for mountings, recommended in earlier issues of this manual, is now discouraged.

Whether the adhesive used is dry mounting tissue or white casein glue, the area of the paper to be covered by the illustration should be indicated before the mounts are placed by drawing a very light pencil line at the top, or placing a dot at each upper corner. The illustration, or the composite of illustrations, should be centered upon the page. "Centering" in this connection assumes a slightly wider margin at the bottom of the sheet than at the top, and a half-inch wider margin at the left than at the right (to compensate for the visual loss due to the binding).

As each page of mounted material is finished, it should be

set aside to dry for a few minutes (follow precisely the directions for drying mountings made with dry mounting tissue) before being placed under a weight for several hours. It is advisable to protect the newly mounted material by putting a piece of plain paper between each two sheets while they are under a weight.

A word of caution is not out of place to the student who proposes to develop and print his own photographs. The job should not be attempted by an amateur unless all the proper facilities are at hand and, further, unless there is ample time to carry out the successive steps without hurry and to allow for possible accidents. Many a roll of film has been ruined by too little care having been used in washing off the developing agent—to mention but one hazard.

It cannot be emphasized too strongly that sufficient time should be set aside for this job of mounting illustrations. Unless he is cautioned beforehand, the inexperienced person is likely to underestimate grossly the time that is required to do this work satisfactorily.

92. *Folding.*—Illustrations larger than the normal page size may usually be reduced photographically. If reduction is not feasible, as it may not be in the case of large maps, for example, the material may be folded, provided that the institution for which the paper is prepared does not prohibit folding.

To fold, work first from right to left, making the first crease no more than 7½ inches from the left side of the sheet. If a second fold is necessary, carry the right-hand portion of the sheet back to the right, making the second crease no more than 6½ inches to the left of the first. Additional folds, if required, should be parallel with the first two. If the folding is done as directed, when the large folded sheet is in place, there will be no danger of the folds at the left being caught in the stitching or of those at the right being sheared off in the process of trimming. Folding in more than one direction should be avoided, but, if it is not possible to do so, the sheet should first be folded from bottom to top, making the first fold no more than 10 inches from the top of the sheet. When this first fold has been made, a strip 1 inch wide should be cut from the upper portion of the sheet (i.e., the portion that has been folded up), along the left edge, from the top down to the bottom fold. The removal of this strip is necessary to prevent the free portion of the sheet from being caught in the stitching. The folding from right to left should be as directed above.

93. *Numbering of pages.*—Pages of illustrative materials should be numbered consecutively with the textual matter. It is not permissible to insert them after the text has been numbered by giving them supplementary numbers (e.g., 45*a*). A folded sheet is numbered in the center at the top of the exposed fold.

XII

Appendix

94. The appendix stands in somewhat the same relation to the paper as content footnotes in that it provides a place for material that is not absolutely necessary to the text. In it may be placed tables too detailed for text presentation; technical notes on method, and schedules and forms used in collecting materials; copies of documents not generally available to the reader; case studies too long to be put into text; and sometimes illustrative materials. If the materials thus relegated to an appendix are numerous in each of several categories, each category should form a separate appendix. Thus the appendixes would be numbered or lettered (I, II, etc., or A, B, etc.).

Assigning titles to the appendixes is at the discretion of the writer, but if one is titled, all must be.

Spacing depends upon the nature of the material and need not be the same for all the appendixes. Documents and case studies may well be in single space, whereas explanations of methods and procedures, which are possibly referred to more often, are more easily read in double space—or in space and one-half if that is used in the main body of the paper.

Appendix I

Typing the Paper

ADVANCE PREPARATIONS

95. *The writer's responsibility for editing.*—Before final typing, the writer should edit the paper. He alone is responsible for the correct presentation of the content and the reference and illustrative materials. The editing will save his time if he expects to do the typing himself, and it will save unnecessary errors, which would require correction in the final copy, involving both time and expense.

Beyond the production of an accurate transcription of the copy, the typist should be held responsible only for mechanical details having to do with neatness, spacing, and the general appearance of the final copy.

96. *Typewriter.*—Either pica or elite type, or one of the types available on some of the newer models, is satisfactory for most typing jobs, although some institutions specify pica type for theses and dissertations. A typist who expects to do any considerable amount of typing of theses, dissertations, or other formal papers —particularly those designed for submission to publishers— would do well to provide herself with a specially equipped typewriter, preferably with pica type. The special vertical spacing obtainable with the five-line ratchet is recommended for the typing of copy that is to be reproduced by planographing (also called lithoprinting), and it may be used for any other copy, subject to the approval of the person for whom the copy is to be prepared. The same ratchet permits single and double spacing, and the accurate half-space turn of the roller is a great convenience in the typing of superscripts and subscripts. Keys with the grave accent mark (`), the acute accent mark (´), the plus symbol (+), the plus-and-minus symbol (±), and the square brackets ([]) are almost indispensable. Some of the symbols carried on the standard keyboard are used less frequently in the typing of formal papers than in commercial work and can be replaced with the more necessary symbols at a nominal charge. Some typewriters now available have certain keys that are designed for easy removal and replacement with others. The manufacturers stock a wide variety of characters and will make others to order at reasonable prices.

Both type and rollers should be kept clean by the use of a specially treated paper. After placing the typewriter in stencil position, the special paper is inserted and each key is struck firmly five or six times, or until the impression leaves no ink smudge. The rollers are cleaned during the typing operation. Periodically, a thorough check of the typewriter should be made by a responsible serviceman to insure smooth rollers, uniformity of letter impression, alignment of letters, and proper adjustment of tension.

97. *Ribbon.*—Ribbons of superior quality are most satisfactory in the long run. Medium-inked black ribbons produce greater uniformity of impression than the light-inked or the heavy-inked. To secure superior uniformity of type color, it is desirable to have on hand before the typing is begun enough ribbons of the same kind to complete the job, and to rotate them at regular intervals of, say, every twenty-five pages. This is particularly desirable in typing copy for planographing.

98. *Paper.*—A good grade of bond paper should be used. Do not use one of the so-called erasable papers, unless it is specified by the institution to which the paper is to be presented. Some institutions have specific requirements for theses and dissertations. If there are no such requirements, paper of 20-pound weight and at least 50 per cent rag content should be used. Some institutions permit a lighter weight for the carbon copies.

99. *Carbon paper.*—The carbon paper should be of good quality: black, hard finish (non-greasy), light- or medium-weight (light-weight is preferable if several copies are to be made). Such carbon paper makes a gray rather than a black impression, but the letters are sharper, and the copies smudge less and remain in good condition longer than those made with paper of a soft or medium finish.

The use of carbon paper on which the lines are numbered in a vertical column visible at the right of the typing paper is preferred by some typists to the guide sheet mentioned below (sec. 112, p. 137).

MECHANICS OF TYPING

100. *Spacing.*—The text should be typed either double space or space and one-half (sec. 96). Rules for spacing are given in the context of other matters of style as they relate to quotations (pp. 16-17), footnotes (pp. 137-39), bibliography (p. 72), tables (p. 111), illustrations (pp. 118, 121), and appendix (p. 126), and also in the sections concerned with table of contents (pp. 132-33), list of tables (p. 133), list of illustrations (p. 134), subheadings (p. 135), beginning new pages (p. 134), and punctuation (p. 130).

101. *Spacing after punctuation.*—Leave one space after commas and semicolons; two spaces after colons, except when they are used in scriptural references and in separating hours and minutes (e.g., Rom. 8:14-20, 4:30 P.M.); two spaces after exclamation marks, question marks, and periods ending sentences. Do not space after the first period in such abbreviations as i.e., e.g., A.M., P.M. (likewise a.m. and p.m.), A.D., B.C., U.S., N.Y., B.A., M.S., Ph.D., N.B.C., B.B.C.; but do leave a space between the periods and the initials of the name of a person, as, for example, J. R. C. Stewart. Distinguish between a hyphen and a dash: Leave no space before or after a hyphen ("fast-growing city"); make a dash by typing two hyphens without space between them or at either end (e.g., "This kind of education, while it may--in fact, does--very well meet . . .").

102. *Margins.*—Leave a margin of at least one inch on each of the four sides of the sheet. Some institutions require more than this, particularly on the left, since binding reduces the margin. On the first page of every major division of the paper (see sec. 108, p. 134), leave two inches at the top above the heading (i.e., begin typing on the twelfth line from the top).

103. *Indention.*—Indent paragraphs six to eight spaces, unless specific regulations are made. Follow the same scheme of paragraph indention consistently.

104. *Pagination.*—Assign a number to every page except the blank sheet following the title page. On the title page—and the half-title pages, if there are any—the numbers are not shown.

   a) For the preliminaries, number with small Roman numerals (i, ii, iv, etc.) centered at the bottom of the page on the fifth space above the edge. The numbering begins with "ii"; the title page counts as page i.

b) Number the remaining parts, including text, illustrations, appendix, and bibliography with Arabic numerals, centered at the top of the page on the fifth space below the edge, except that on every page with a major heading (e.g., the first page of a chapter, of the bibliography, etc.), place the number at the foot of the page, centered on the fifth space above the edge. Begin the numbering of the main body of the paper with "1" and run consecutively to the end.

An alternate scheme of pagination is that of numbering all pages in the upper right-hand corner—excepting of course the title page and half-title pages.

105. *Table of contents.*—Tables of contents vary widely both in style and in the amount of information included. For some papers, listing of chapters alone is considered adequate, except that any introduction, appendix, or bibliography should be included. For some, a more or less complete outline may be desirable. But for the greater number, something between the two extremes is usually best. Subdivisions may be omitted—all of them or only those of lower levels. When included, however, they should appear in the order of their rank. It is not suitable, for example, to express first-level subheadings and then to skip to a third- or fourth-level, or to begin with any but the first level. All chapter titles, and subdivision titles if any, must agree exactly with their wording in the body of the paper. Ordinarily, the preliminaries are not included in the contents, but sometimes they are, especially the preface.

Three styles of contents are shown in Appendix III (pp. 152-54). Sample A illustrates in general a style suited to the needs of the average paper. Separation into parts, to be sure, is by no means average practice. But parts as well as chapters are included in Sample A in order to show their proper expression in type style and spacing.

Looking at Sample A, notice that

a) Heading is centered on the twelfth line from the top of the page.

b) Headings of parts are centered above the chapters they include.

c) All major headings are typed in capital letters throughout.

d) All subheadings are typed in capital and small letters. (If lower levels of subdivisions are also shown, they are usually typed in small letters except for the first word, proper nouns, and proper adjectives.)

e) Chapter numbers, here shown in Roman numerals ending with a period, are so aligned that the longest number will begin at the margin. If Arabic rather than Roman numerals are used at the heads of chapters, they are of course used in the Contents.

f) The word "Chapter" stands at the head of the column of chapter numbers (actually, the inclusion of "Chapter" is optional). It is omitted if the chapters are not formally so called.

g) Vertical spacing is as follows: *Triple* between TABLE OF CONTENTS and first entry, and between PART and preceding entry. *Double* between PART and the following entry, between chapter headings, and between chapter headings and the *first* entry of a subdivision. *Single* between individual subheadings.

h) A heading of such length that it would extend beyond the point of the last period leader is divided and the runover aligned vertically with the preceding part.

i) Chapter headings begin on the third space after the period following the chapter number.

j) Subheadings are indented three spaces from major headings. (If more than one level of subdivision is shown, each *level* is indented three spaces from that of the preceding higher level.)

k) Period leaders connect major headings with their appropriate page numbers. Their use with subheadings depends on page numbers being shown. Leaders stop at the third space (at least) preceding the first digit of the longest page number. Period leaders must always be aligned vertically.

m) Page numbers are so placed that the last digit is next to the right-hand margin.

Samples B and C illustrate two styles of contents, either one of which may be suitable when a single level of subdivision is to be shown. The units may be separated with dashes, semicolons, or periods. If page numbers are included, they are usually placed within parentheses and preceding the mark of punctuation separating the units.

This style is especially appropriate when there are many short first-level subheadings. It is sometimes used as well when an analysis is considered desirable in the table of contents even though the subheadings are not expressed in the text.

If a table of contents must be carried over to a second page (or more), so apportion the material that in general a major heading with its subheadings appears on the same page. An exception may be made when the complete chapter unit is long, but in no case should a major heading be placed at the foot of a page with fewer than two lines of subheading beneath it. Begin the continuation on the sixth line from the top of the page and omit any heading (i.e., omit TABLE OF CONTENTS —CONTINUED or CONTINUED).

If a table of contents occupies less than a page, the entire body of typed matter should be approximately centered vertically upon the page. (See sec. 91, p. 123, for an interpretation of centering.) The heading, however, should never be set higher than the twelfth line from the top of the page, and the space between the final entry and the bottom of the sheet should never be less than one inch.

106. *List of tables.*—As reference to the sample in Appendix III shows (see p. 155), this list is essentially in the same style as the table of contents. The heading appears on the twelfth line (or lower, if the list is short) from the top. The table headings,

agreeing exactly with their expression above the tables themselves, are typed in capital and small letters. Period leaders connect titles with page numbers.

107. *List of illustrations.*—If the paper includes both plates and figures and they are few in number, both may be shown in the
list of illustrations, each group under its appropriate subheading. Plate numbers are normally in capital Roman numerals,
figure numbers in Arabic. Period leaders connect titles with
page numbers. The titles of plates should agree with those given
on the plates themselves; but when the legends beneath the figures are long, a shortened form in the list of illustrations is usually permissible. For a thesis or a dissertation, however, checking with the dissertations department is advisable. If a descriptive or explanatory statement in addition to the title appears with
the illustration, that statement should be omitted from the list.
(A sample list of illustrations is shown in Appendix III, p. 155.)

108. *Major headings beginning new pages.*—Begin every major
division (i.e., preface, contents, list of tables, list of illustrations,
introduction, each new chapter, bibliography, appendix) on a
new page. Center the heading in capital letters on the twelfth
line from the top of the sheet. If the paper is divided into sections
termed "chapters," the chapter number appears alone (e.g.,
"CHAPTER I") on the twelfth line, and the chapter title is centered on the third line beneath it. If chapter is not formally
expressed and the sections are merely numbered, the number
and title (e.g., "I. THE WORLD OF 1815") are centered on
the twelfth line. If the title is longer than 48 spaces, set it in two
(or more) double-spaced lines, in inverted-pyramid form. Use
no punctuation at the ends of lines. Begin typing the text or the
first entry of a list (contents, etc.), on the third line below the
heading.

109. *Subheadings.*—Because of their bearing on the organization of the text, subheadings in their various forms and the order in which they should be employed are discussed in the chapter on the text (see sec. 10, pp. 5-6).

Type centered subheadings in capital and small letters, and all other subheadings in small letters except for the first word, proper nouns, and proper adjectives. A centered subheading of more than 48 spaces should be divided into two or more single-spaced lines, in inverted-pyramid form. A side heading of more than a half-line should be divided more or less evenly into two (or more) single-spaced lines, the runovers beginning at the margin. Paragraph headings should be underlined and should end with a period and a dash (two hyphens). All other subheadings should omit punctuation at the ends of lines.

All subheadings begin on the third space below text. If two (or more) subheadings appear together (i.e., without intervening text), a double space should be left between them, and a double space left also between the subheading and the text following.

110. *Corrections and erasures.*—No interlineations, crossing out of letters or words, strikeovers, or extensive erasures are permissible. Deletion or addition of more than one letter after the line has been completed should be made by retyping. By skillful use of the back-spacer, the letters of a word can be crowded so that the space normally occupied by a word of given length can be made to accommodate a word having one more letter. This must be done by erasing the entire word and reducing evenly the space between the letters, not by crowding just two letters. Extensive correction of a page once passed calls for great care in retyping so that the material may be equalized and the last line on the page properly spaced out to the end. Erasures should be reduced to a minimum and made with such skill on both the original and the copies that they will not be noticeable. Wherever possible they should be made before the page is removed from the typewriter. Typists should form the habit of looking over each page before removing it from the machine. Once withdrawn, each copy of the set should be corrected separately by direct type rather than all together by restacking and insertion of carbons. Care should be exercised to strike the keys heavily or lightly, as the case may require, so that the corrected portions may match in color as nearly as possible the remainder of the typed material upon the page.

An erasing shield and two ink erasers—one with a broad edge for covering larger areas and one with a narrow edge for the smaller ones—are indispensable. To prevent smudging of the face copy, the fingers should rest on the erasing shield. To prevent smudging of the carbon copies, a piece of paper should be placed between each sheet of carbon and the page beneath.

Corrections on copy prepared for planographing must not be made by erasing. The use of a chemically treated paper such as KO-REC-TYPE (for the face copy) and KO-REC-COPY (for carbon copy) will remove mistakes in typing both on the original and the carbon copy (or copies) in one easy operation. This is especially helpful in correcting copy that is to be planographed, but it may of course be used in all typing. If errors on copy for planographing are not corrected in that way, the corrected word or words should be retyped on a separate piece of paper and placed over the errors, attaching with a light coating of rubber cement. Great care must be taken to place the patch accurately and neatly and to leave no dark lines or specks which would show in the printed copy. Typing the corrections on white gummed paper is an alternative to typing on plain paper and pasting.

TYPING THE FOOTNOTES

111. *Spacing, indention, footnote numeral.*—Separate text and foot-notes with an unbroken line twenty spaces in length, beginning at the left-hand margin on the first line beneath the text. The first line of footnote material is on the second line below this (the third line under the text). Indent the first line of each foot-note the same number of spaces as the paragraph indention in the text. Type the footnotes single space, but use double space between individual notes.

Place the footnote numeral slightly above the line (never a full space above). There should be no punctuation after the numeral and no extra space between it and the first of the note.

[1]G. D. H. Cole, Self-government in Industry, p. 16.

112. *Estimating space for text and footnotes.*—To place the foot-notes correctly on the page and maintain the proper margin at the foot of the page, a *guide sheet* should be used. A special car-bon paper may be used (see sec. 99, p. 129) or a sheet may be made of firm, light-weight wrapping paper. Cut it the same length as the typing paper and one-half inch wider. Measure off top and bottom margins to correspond with those used on the typed page, insert the paper into the typewriter, and, begin-ning with "1" on the line with that occupied by the first line of text on the typed page, number down the extreme right-hand edge of the guide sheet to the line opposite that of the last line of typed matter. It is helpful also to indicate in the top and bot-tom margins of the guide sheet the point opposite which the page number should appear (see sec. 104, pp. 130-31).

Before rolling the paper and guide sheet into the typewriter, place the guide sheet beneath the bottom sheet of typing paper;

align the top and left-hand edges of paper, carbon paper, and guide sheet so that the numbered edge of the guide sheet extends beyond the typing paper; and roll the stacked paper into the typewriter. It may be necessary to adjust the top edges after the paper is placed in the machine.

When the first footnote number appears in the text, stop and count the number of lines in the corresponding footnote, add two to allow for the line of separation, and deduct this total from the total number of type lines as shown on the guide sheet. The difference between the two figures will give the number of the line at the end of which to stop typing text in order to allow proper space for the footnote. As each succeeding footnote number appears in the text, add the number of lines in the corresponding footnote, allowing one extra for the space between notes, and again determine the number of text lines to be typed.

All will go according to plan, and the bottom margin will be the proper depth unless a footnote number occurs in the last line of text after all available footnote space has been allotted. Make it a habit to look ahead so as to discover such a difficulty, and avoid the necessity of retyping the page by omitting the last line, even though this will result in a bottom margin deeper than usual.

A similar difficulty arises when a footnote number shows the corresponding footnote to be longer than can be accommodated in the space remaining on the page. This calls for a division of the footnote.

113. *Continuation of a long footnote to the following page.*—Begin the note on the page where reference to it appears in the text and type as much as the page will allow, taking care to break the note within a sentence. Carry the remainder into the footnote area of the next page, where it precedes the footnotes for that page. To indicate the continuation of a foonote by such a statement as "Continued on the next page" is bad form.

114. *Arrangement of short footnotes.*—To avoid the unattractive appearance and the waste of space which result from the placement of many short footnotes, each on a line by itself and separated from its fellows by extra space above and below, it is advisable to let such short notes follow each other on the same line. There must, however, be at least three spaces between notes, and *all the notes on one line must be complete*. It is not permissible to carry over to the next line a part of the last note. Similarly, it is not permissible to utilize the blank space following a note of more than one line in length to insert a short note.

Wrong: [1]John Dove, Confutation of Atheism, p. 125. [2]Ibid., pp. 128-29.

Wrong: [1]G. D. H. Cole, Self-government in Industry (5th ed. rev.; London: G. Bell & Co., 1920), p. 2. [2]Ibid., p. 9.

115. *Arrangement of footnotes on a short page.*—If for any reason a page containing footnotes cannot be typed to full measure, the footnotes should be arranged at the bottom of the page, not immediately below the text. This rule need not apply, however, to the final page of a chapter.

116. *Arrangement of footnotes included in a quotation.*—When a single-spaced, indented quotation includes one or more footnote reference indexes, the corresponding footnotes should be placed beneath the quotation, separated from the last line of the quotation by an eight-space rule. Thus the identical reference indexes appearing in the quotation are retained and it is made clear to the reader that the notes are part of the material quoted.

Appendix II

Some Rules of Punctuation

117. Punctuation in what may be called its secondary use has been treated to some extent in all the preceding chapters.[1] Here, for the benefit of those who may desire to review the subject, it will be briefly dealt with in its relation to sentence structure. The matters discussed are mainly those that for the most part students seem to understand the least and therefore to overlook the most often.

118. *Period*

    a) A period should be placed at the end of a complete declarative or imperative sentence, and although in compound sentences two or more subject-predicate elements may be separated by semicolons (see "Semicolon," below), the substitution of a comma, as in the following, is a common fault:

<u>Wrong:</u> The hour was late, we were obliged to go by automobile.

    b) Commas may be properly used, however, to separate independent clauses that are closely connected in thought, especially when they not only have the same subject but employ the same tense.

He was fitted by education and training, he had no close family ties, he was fired by a sense of mission.

---

[1] This section is based on the rules set forth in *A Manual of Style*.

Also, very short sentences closely connected in thought may use commas to separate the clauses.

```
John is going to Europe, Debby is going to Maine, I am going to
school.
```

119. *Colon*

a) A colon marks the point at which the idea expressed in one clause is followed by another clause or by a phrase (or more) that expands, clarifies, or exemplifies its meaning.

```
There was another result no less inevitable:  all they knew must
be kept jealously within the organization.
```

```
There are, first, two functions to be considered:  its signifi-
cance as a repository and its significance as an instrument of
research.
```

b) A colon is placed at the end of a grammatical element introducing a formal statement, whether the statement is quoted or not. It is always placed after "following," "as follows," "thus," "in sum," and the like.

```
He summed it up thus:  "Our capital is intellectual; . . . "
```

```
And, finally:  There can be no question, in view of the evidence
presented, that the man committed a forgery.
```

```
His "laws" are as follows:  books are for use; every reader his
book; . . .
```

120. *Semicolon*

a) A semicolon is used between parts of a compound sentence that are not connected by a conjunction. Note that the following adverbs (and there are others) should not be treated like conjunctions, but should be preceded by semicolons, not commas: "consequently," "hence," "however," "indeed," "therefore," "thus," "yet."

```
In India the idea of truth became completely separated from out-
side fact; hence all outside was illusion; truth was an inner
disposition.
```

It recognizes that men's judgments and conclusions about space
are purely of his own making; yet we need to recognize . . .

b) A semicolon may be used to separate independent clauses
that are closely connected in thought.

Let us grant the evils of vicarious living; let us also grant
its necessity.

c) When any of the elements in a series contains a comma, the
units are separated by semicolons.

Three cities that have had notable success with the program are
Hartford, Connecticut; Kalamazoo, Michigan; and Pasadena, California.

The percentages of failures were as follows: Class A, 7 per
cent; Class B, 13 per cent; and Class C, 30 per cent.

121. *Comma.*—Although the comma indicates the smallest inter-
ruption in continuity of thought or sentence structure, when it
is correctly used it does more for ease of reading and ready un-
derstanding than any mark of punctuation.

a) Used in pairs, commas set off elements that are actually
parenthetic in nature. If one of the pair is omitted, part of
the parenthetic matter is run into a clause or phrase to which
it does not belong, thus producing a sentence that is awk-
ward in its association of ideas and difficult to read. No one
should be guilty of sentences punctuated like the following:

Wrong: John Ross, 24 was among the missing.

Wrong: My mother, who lives in New York spent the winter in
Florida.

Wrong: The bill you will be pleased to hear, passed at the
last session.

b) Ordinarily, put a comma between independent clauses
joined by "and," "but," "or," "nor," or "for" when there is
a change of subject.

This was an ancient custom among the Greeks, and the Romans took
it over from them.

He would glorify the victor so far as he was really glorious,
but other men would "tell a tale decked out with dazzling lies."

c) The comma should be omitted, however, in short sentences
composed of clauses closely connected in thought.

He arrived at noon and I took him directly to the meeting.

d) A comma may be used to separate short independent clauses
that are closely connected in thought when they have the
same subject and employ the same tense.

He was fitted by education and training, he had no close family
ties, he was fired by a sense of mission.

e) When two grammatical elements that are not independent
clauses are joined by "and," "but," "or," "nor," use no
comma between them.

This was accomplished by assisting the pupil to clarify her
thought and to relate clearly one part of it to another.

f) Use commas to set off a non-restrictive clause or phrase;
omit them around a restrictive clause or phrase. An element
is non-restrictive if it is not essential to the meaning of the
main clause and may be omitted. A clause or phrase is restrictive when it is needed to identify the word it modifies.

These books, which are placed on reserve in the Library, are required reading for the course. [The clause is non-restrictive,
since the meaning of the main clause, "These books are required
reading for the course," is unchanged if the parenthetical
clause is omitted.]

The books which are required reading for the course are placed
on reserve in the library. [Here the clause is restrictive; it
identifies the books placed on reserve as those that are "required reading for the course."]

The deserted mill, standing with idle wheel beside the rushing
stream, marked the spot where the road turned toward the lake.
[Non-restrictive.]

The building standing on the site of the old courthouse is the
newest in the business section. [Restrictive.]

g) Separate with commas two or more coordinate phrases or clauses ending in a word that governs or modifies another word in a following clause or phrase.

```
She both delighted in, and was disturbed by, her new leisure and
freedom.
```

```
It is a logical, if as I fear a harsh, solution to the problem.
```

h) Use a comma to separate an opening subordinate clause or an adverbial phrase, or an introductory phrase containing a gerund, participle, or infinitive from the main clause.

```
Although he had never been on a pack trip, he agreed to go.
```

```
As far as mechanics of presentation are concerned, one can un-
derstand . . .
```

```
If that is correct, they have no reason for complaint.
```

```
Hoping that his fellows would soon catch up with him, he stopped
to rest.
```

i) Set off with commas words or phrases that make a distinct break in the flow of thought.

```
This statement, therefore, cannot be verified.
```

```
However, the motion was tabled.
```

```
That, after all, is not a matter of great importance.
```

j) But omit the comma with such words when the connection is close and the sentence reads smoothly.

```
It is therefore clear that the deposits were made . . .
```

```
He was perhaps thinking of the future.
```

```
The deception was indeed obvious.
```

k) Use commas to set off a noun or a phrase that is in apposition to another noun.

His brother, a Harvard graduate, transferred to Princeton for his work in theology.

A one-time officer in the Foreign Legion, the man hoped to escape further military duty.

m) If, however, the appositive limits the meaning of the noun, no commas should be used.

The Danish philosopher Kierkegaard once wrote: "What is anxiety?"

The motion picture <u>Becket</u> is adapted from the play by Jean Anouilh.

n) A series of three or more words, phrases, or clauses should be separated by commas, even though the last in the series is preceded by "and."

New York, Chicago, and Los Angeles were the cities mentioned.

He asserted that dishes had been broken, cutlery lost, and carpets and upholstery soiled beyond the possibility of renovation.

o) Set off contrasted elements with commas.

The idea, not its expression, is significant.

The harder we run, the more we stand in the same place.

p) Use a comma to separate two identical or closely similar words.

They marched in, in twos.

Whatever is, had better be accepted.

q) Although adjectives in a series are normally separated by commas, if the last adjective is more closely connected to the noun than are the others, omit the comma between the last two adjectives.

At the intersection is a large, new brick house.

He was a ragged, spindly little fellow.

r) A comma is used to prevent misreading of such sentences as the following:

```
Of Grant, Lincoln said . . .

After eating, the lions yawned and then dozed.

Outside, the house appeared larger than the size of the rooms
indicated.
```

s) Do not use a comma between the two parts of a compound predicate.

```
Those men fell in love with the American wilderness and learned
its contour and moods.
```

122. *Dash.*—Dashes are used to set off material that is parenthetic or summary in nature. In typing, distinguish between a dash and a hyphen. A dash consists of two hyphens without space either between them or at either side.

```
He arrived late--a circumstance I should have mentioned earlier.
```

a) Use dashes to mark an interpolation or a sudden break in thought causing a change in sentence structure.

```
In the Sermon on the Mount--the style of the New Testament is,
of course, formed on that of the Old--occurs this passage.

And yet--here is the Greek miracle--this absolute simplicity of
structure is alone in majesty of beauty . . .

To this the young man answered--he must have been very young--
"I will do as you say."
```

b) Introduce by a dash an element that emphasizes or explains the main clause through repetition of a key-word.

```
But where shall wisdom be found?--the wisdom that is above ru-
bies. [When it is needed, an interrogation point or an exclama-
tion point may be inserted before the dash in a sentence like
this.]
```

c) Dashes should be used to set off the insertion of a defining or enumerating element, or the addition of a summary, whether the summary is a clause, a phrase, or a simple list.

The English House of Lords, endowed with all the best the world could give--power, riches, reverential respect--fought with all her might . . .

The statue of the man throwing the discus, the charioteer at Delphi, the stern young horsemen of the Parthenon frieze, and the poetry of Pinder--all show the culmination of the great ideal . . .

Each student kept a record of everything he read--good, bad, and indifferent.

123. *Hyphen.*—A hyphen is used to join two or more words which in combination form a single term—a compound word. Many such words are familiar (e.g., "twenty-one," "two-thirds," "by-product"); many more may not be, and a dictionary is of little help, especially as writers constantly coin new compounds to fit their needs. For a thorough treatment of the subject, *A Manual of Style* should be consulted. Selected from the *Manual* and commented upon below are some of the more common usages.

a) Hyphenate phrases used as adjectives when the word combinations formed might be ambiguous.

high-school course	well-known man
first-class investment	better-trained teachers
nineteenth-century progress	English-speaking peoples

house-to-house canvass
two-year-old boy
much-needed rest

b) However, many word-combinations requiring hyphens when placed before a noun are not hyphenated when they are used after the word modified.

He is a man well known for his interest in civic affairs.

The new salary scale should attract teachers who are better trained.

The company's accounting methods are strictly up to date.

c) Hyphenate combinations of (1) noun or adjective with a participle, or (2) present participle with a preposition that does not govern the noun following.

dark-colored	liquor-crazed	war-marred
dog-tired	sinister-looking	lean-to
foreign-born	quiet-spoken	leveling-up

d) Use hyphens in compounds the last term of which is derived from a transitive verb.

clay-modeling	pleasure-loving	noun-coinage
labor-saving	hero-worship	office-holder
information-seeking	pain-killer	wage-earner

e) In general, use hyphens with the prefixes "all-," "ex-," "self-," "vice-," and with the suffix "-elect."

all-embracing	ex-president	self-rule	governor-elect
all-knowing	ex-serviceman	self-made	senator-elect

vice-regent
(But: viceroy)

f) Omit the hyphen in compounds the first term of which is derived from a verb.

boarding school	meeting place	trading post
flying field	running board	turning point
boiling point	rocking chair	whipping boy

g) Use no hyphen for a combination the first word of which is an adverb ending with "-ly," or for a combination of adverb and participle when no ambiguity would result (since an adverb cannot modify a noun).

easily found answer	slightly elevated walk
readily recognized principle	heavily populated area
ever increasing interest	evenly distributed wealth

h) In general, prefixes when joined to roots drop the hyphen except when

(1) joined to a proper noun or a proper adjective;

```
pre-Cambrian
Pan-Islamic
un-Christian
```

(2) joined to a word with a first vowel that would form a diphthong with the last vowel of the prefix;

```
co-author
co-worker
ante-urban
```

(3) absence of the hyphen would suggest mispronunciation, or would confuse the word with one of a different meaning.

```
pre-eminent
re-cover [to cover again]
re-create [to create again]
```

But for the following—to mention but a few—no hyphen is used between the prefix and the root.

```
biweekly            prehistoric              rearrange
coeducation         prewar                   reword
coexistent          overconfident            unhandy
```

i) Hyphenate compounds denoting equal participation.

```
author-critic        city-state              soldier-statesman
```

j) When a compound word, the last of a series, is preceded by others of the same base word represented only by a modifier in each case, a hyphen should be placed after each modifier.

```
All over Greece there were games and athletic contests:  horse-,
boat-, foot-, torch-races among them.
```

```
The six- and seven-year-olds were assigned first- and second-
grade lessons.
```

k) Hyphenate such adjectival compounds as the following:

```
do-it-yourself kit            every-other-year arrangement
go-as-you-please fashion      now-or-never choice
```

124. *Parentheses.*—It has been pointed out that some matter that is parenthetic in nature is set off with commas and some other with dashes. Still other, less relevant to the main argument than clauses and phrases set off with commas and dashes, is enclosed in parentheses.

```
I (being the person least concerned) could conveniently take an-
other train.
```

```
The coverage seems complete (I will enlarge upon this in the
next section).
```

The more common uses of parentheses are discussed and illustrated in earlier chapters.

125. *Brackets*
   a) Any interpolation into a quotation by the writer using the quotation must be enclosed in brackets (see *h*, pp. 24-25).
   b) Parenthetical matter within a parenthesis is enclosed in brackets.

```
The book is available in translation (see J. R. Evans-Wentz, The
Tibetan Book of the Dead [Oxford:  Oxford University Press,
1927]).
```

   c) If further parenthesis within the bracket is required, use parentheses again.

```
The various arguments advanced (these include certain anonymous
writers [Public Economy (New York, 1848)]) may be formulated
thus: . . .
```

126. *Quotation marks and ellipsis marks.*—These are discussed at some length in the chapter on "Quotations" (secs. 18 *d*), *e*), pp. 17-19; *g*), pp. 20-24).

127. *Punctuation marks with parentheses,*
   brackets, and quotation marks
   a) The punctuation of a sentence containing either a paren-

thetic or a bracketed element depends upon the grammatical nature both of the matter outside and the matter inside the parentheses (or brackets). If the parenthetic (bracketed) matter is an independent sentence, it is given the appropriate terminal punctuation (see n. 1 below), and the element preceding it is also punctuated as its nature requires. If it calls for a comma, semicolon, or dash, the mark is transferred to follow the parenthesis (n. 1); if a colon, it is placed before or after the parenthesis as the structure and meaning may dictate; if a period, question mark, or exclamation mark, it must be placed before the parenthesis, since in such case the parenthetic element is not closely joined to it either in thought or in grammatical structure (see n. 2). If, however, the entire unit ends after the parenthesis, the period follows the final parenthesis (see n. 3).

[1]Thus a novel is not analyzed, . . . until we have discovered its place in the mind of the novelist (is this the "intentional fallacy"?), in the movement of the age, . . .

[2]Quotations from the French novels are translated for the reader by the author. (Are the "bourgeois épanouis" in the country fair scene in Madame Bovary "expansive bourgeois"?)

[3]The archduke had his own audience, privy council, and council of state (along with lesser bodies).

The rules just mentioned do not apply to parentheses enclosing figures or letters marking enumerations.

b) Rules for the placing of other marks of punctuation when they occur at the point of the final quotation mark are as follows. Periods and commas are always placed inside quotation marks; semicolons and colons, outside. Question marks and exclamation marks are placed outside the quotation marks unless the question or the exclamation occurs within the matter quoted (see subsec. f, pp. 19-20).

Appendix III

Sample Pages of a Paper

Three styles of tables of contents are shown here: one in which the paper is divided into parts as well as into chapters (see sec. 105, p. 131) and two in which the subheadings are run in plain paragraph (*ibid.*, p. 133). Only a part of the contents is shown in each sample.

[Sample A]

TABLE OF CONTENTS

[Sample B]

CONTENTS

Aim of the book; Leonardo's boyhood; apprenticeship to
Verrocchio; Verrocchio's painting and sculpture; Leonardo's part in Verrocchio's Baptism; the Uffizzi Annunciation; the Liechtenstein portrait; the Munich Madonna;
the Benois Madonna; the Louvre Annunciation

The Uffizi Adoration; Leonardo's departure to Milan; his
engines of war; the list of his works; the Vatican St.
Jerome; the Paris Virgin of the Rocks; the portraits;
Leonardo's pupils; Leonardo and Salai

[Sample C]

CONTENTS

Romanticism (1)--Nationalism (3)--Liberalism (6)--The
Industrial Revolution (11)

The Problem (14)--France (15)--Germany (16)--Prussia and
Austria as Reconstituted at Vienna (18)--Italy, the "Geographical Expression" (24)--The Other Countries (26)

The Holy Alliance (27)--The Quadruple Alliance (30)--Dip-
lomatic Congresses (33)--Uprisings in Spain and Naples (36)
--Alliance System and the Monroe Doctrine (39)--Greek Re-
volt (42)--Belgian Revolution of 1830 (44)

LIST OF TABLES

LIST OF ILLUSTRATIONS[1]

[1] The list of illustrations should be placed on a separate page from the list of tables.

[Sample: First page of a chapter, showing chapter number dropped to the twelfth space from the upper edge of the paper. The text is double spaced; the "long quotations" and the footnotes are single spaced.]

CHAPTER I

THE DEVELOPMENT OF A RACE RELATIONS

ACTION-STRUCTURE

Race Relations in the British Isles
1700 to World War I

A small Negro population was living in London by 1700, and some sources have estimated that by 1770 there were between 14,000 and 20,000 Negroes residing in greater London out of a total population of some 123,000.[1] They were mainly slaves and domestic servants living in white homes, and of their relations with whites of their own class, one student has written:

> . . . colour sensibility as such was very little in evidence. . . . No doubt Negroes in general were thought of more as slaves and servants than anything else, but there appears to have been no aversion to meeting or mixing with a person simply on the ground of his colour.[2]

During this same period there were about 10,000 Irish and 20,000 Jews in London. Hostility toward them was great, and one student has said,

> All foreigners in London who had an outlandish look were likely to be roughly treated, or at least abused, by the mob. The Jews were very unpopular. . . . Jew baiting became a sport, like cock-throwing or bull baiting, or pelting some poor wretch in the pillory.[3]

---

[1] This would be about the same percentage as Negroes constitute of the Chicago population of 1954. Little cites these estimates (Kenneth L. Little, Negroes in Britain, A Study of Racial Relations in English Society [London: Kegan Paul, Trench, Trubner and Co., Ltd., 1947], p. 170), but notes that C. M. Macinnes, in England and Slavery (London: Arrowsmith, 1934), "doubts if the total slave population in England ever rose above 15,000 or at most 20,000."

[2] Little, Negroes in Britain, p. 203.

[3] M. Dorothy George, London Life in the XVIIIth Century (New York: Alfred A. Knopf, 1926), p. 132.

3

Index